HV 245 S65 1990

DATE DUE

DEC 1 5 1992 5313	
DEC 0 6 1994	

BRODART, INC   Cat. No. 23-221

The Sociology of the Caring Professions

The Sociology of the Caring Professions

Edited by
Pamela Abbott and Claire Wallace
Polytechnic South West, Plymouth

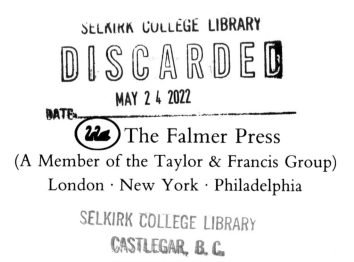

The Falmer Press
(A Member of the Taylor & Francis Group)
London · New York · Philadelphia

UK   The Falmer Press, Rankine Road, Basingstoke, Hampshire, RG24 0PR

USA   The Falmer Press, Taylor & Francis Inc., 1900 Frost Road, Suite 101,
Bristol, PA 19007

First published 1990

British Library Cataloguing in Publication Data
The sociology of the caring professions
    1. Welfare services – Sociological perspectives
    I. Abbott, Pamela   II. Wallace, Claire, 1956–
361

    ISBN 1–85000–819–1
    ISBN 1–85000–824–8 (pbk)

Jacket design by Caroline Archer

Typeset in 11/13 Bembo by
Chapterhouse, The Cloisters, Formby L37 3PX

Printed in Great Britain by Burgess Science Press, Basingstoke on paper which has a specified pH value on final paper manufacture of not less than 7.5 and is therefore 'acid free'.

Contents

1
The Sociology of the Caring Professions: An Introduction

Pamela Abbott and Claire Wallace

This book is concerned with developing a sociological perspective on the caring professions. Whilst a number of occupational groups may claim to be members of this group, the articles in this collection focus mainly on nurses and social workers. This is because, arguably, these two occupational groups represent paradigm cases of caring professions who in their work have a primary commitment to care for their clients; personalized care is central to their practice as professionals. The needs of clients are said to take precedence in their work. There is still a feeling, especially with respect to nursing, that the work is vocational, suggesting a selfless dedication to duty and putting the needs of others first — that is, they are occupations imbued with a service ideology (see Lesley Mackay and Maria Lorentzon, Chapters 3 and 5 in this volume). The professional ethos of social work is profoundly 'client centred', with a strong commitment to respect the individual, to be 'non-judgmental', to 'start where the individual is at' and to allow 'client determination'. A key question is of course the extent to which nurses and social workers are in fact able to deliver personalized care to clients. Both are generally employed within bureaucratic organizations and have to adhere to regulations of the agency which might conflict with what are seen as the needs of the client. Social workers have statutory duties which may require them to take actions which may be opposed to the wishes of the clients. Both nurses and social workers tend to work with individualistic theories about the causes of social problems (see David McCallum, Pamela Abbott and Roger Sapsford, Chapters 8 and 9 in this volume) and intervene at the level of the individual. This often means that the root causes of the client's problems — such as poverty, unemployment, bad housing and so on — are beyond the scope of their professional practice. Nursing and social work (in common with other occupations that lay claim to being caring professions such as probation and youth work) share certain characteristics and problems: they all had their origins in nineteenth-century philanthropy and expanded with the advent of the welfare state into what have been termed 'professional' occupations; they are all concerned with the 'human qualities' of clients to a greater or lesser extent; they are created and sustained through the identification of a particular social problem and the treatment developed for it — in other words with the regulation and control of problematical areas of social life. Related to this latter point, they share particular kinds of knowledge base, aspects of which are derived from sociology as well as other social sciences such as psychology (see Roger Sibeon and David McCullum, Chapters 7 and 8 in this volume). They are often termed the 'semi-professions', being situated within state bureaucracies rather than being represented by independent 'collegiate' organizations in the same way as law or medicine, and this is indicative of the rather fragile status which they hold — their status as 'professions' being often disputed. Related to this perhaps is the fact that these are very often seen as careers for women and therefore intersect with gender ideologies in particular ways. Indeed, they still survive with a penumbra of unqualified volunteer helpers surrounding the career professionals.

The idea of a 'profession' emerged from the medieval universities which served to create the professions of law, medicine and the clergy. These three professions still tend to be seen as the ones against which other claims to professional status are measured. They are characterized by the monopolization of particular forms of expertise, the erection of social boundaries around them through entrance qualifications and extended training, and an ideology of public service and altruism — that is, they claim to serve higher goals than mere economic self interest. This professional autonomy is justified by the self-policing mechanisms constructed through their own internal criteria of standards maintained by the profession itself. Thus, to enter medicine requires a lengthy period of study, a pledge to save life, and adherence to standards of practice set by the teaching hospitals and by the professional associations of the medical profession itself. One consequence of these mechanisms is that they provide the basis for political power in the labour market, allowing the bearers of the profession to command higher status and high rewards for their services. However, critics have pointed out that the professions cannot necessarily be relied upon to police themselves effectively, nor to act in the public interest. Moreover, almost no occupation calling itself a 'profession' can meet all of these criteria. On the whole, this approach of listing the characteristics of professions to measure how far different occupations meet them has been rejected as unhelpful, although Maria Lorentzon in this volume (Chapter 5) partially rejects this view. This is because the traits generally seen as delineating a profession are mostly based upon an idealized conception of the characteristics of the archetypal professions — medicine and law. 'Trait theories' thereby give tacit support to the views which those professions project of themselves to the public. They tend to obscure the middle-class nature of codes of ethics and the ways in which the professions also act as agents of social control.

Friedson has suggested that it is more useful to look at the idea of 'professionalism' as used in practice (Friedson, 1986), whilst Parry and Parry (1976) argue that the key question is how occupational groups achieve the status of 'professional' and in the process gain ascendancy over other occupational groups. Developing this analysis, feminists have argued that in the process of upward mobility, the male-dominated professions gain control over and subordinate female-dominated occupations. This is most clearly illustrated in medicine where the medical profession is male-dominated and where in the process of achieving its dominant professional status, the female occupations of nursing, health visiting and midwifery were subordinated (Abbott and Wallace, Chapter 2 in this volume). Indeed, nurses are still fighting to gain recognition of the right to control their work. Johnson (1972) argues from a Marxist perspective that professions form a particular institutionalized form of client control. Their professional status stems from the ignorance of the client as against professional specialist knowledge, thereby rendering clients relatively helpless. Professionals are accepted as 'specialists' and they often have legal backing for this, making their clients socially and economically dependent. In addition, clients are often socially distanced from their advisers in other ways — by social class, ethnicity, educational background and by gender, for example.

Whilst the Marxist critique sees professionals as acting as the agents of the capitalist state, the Right and feminists have both been critical of the way in which professionals exercise power. Illich *et al.* (1977), for example, have argued that professions are disabling — that is, they take away individuals' ability to care for themselves. Whilst the New Right has attacked monopolistic practices and the political power of the professions, it has tended not to question their ability to provide a necessary service. However, they have questioned the role of welfare professionals, especially social workers, arguing that individuals come to rely on them rather than solving their own problems (Minford, 1987). Feminists have been critical of the ways in which professionals use patriarchal ideology to reinforce the subordinate status of women, for example by the assumption (often unstated) that women should prioritize the needs of their husbands and children over their own (Abbott and Wallace, 1990; Abbott and Sapsford, Chapter 9 in this volume; Lorentzon, Chapter 5 in this volume).

Whilst there is considerable dispute as to the relevance of the term 'professional' for nurses and social workers, they have nevertheless been criticized from both the left and the right in much the same way as the 'established' professions. Etzioni (1969) suggested that occupational groups such as nurses and social workers would be categorized as 'semi-professions' because their work is more 'supervised' and 'applied' than the more theoretically informed and autonomous work of the professions. However, this is based on an idealized 'trait model' of the professions — many doctors and solicitors are employed within bureaucratic organizations and their work is also subject to control and sanctioning.

We would suggest that a more fruitful approach is to examine the ways in which occupational groups make claims to be professions and to examine the extent to which they are successful. Both nursing and social work have made such claims: both occupational groups are still striving to demonstrate that caring is work and to find ways of caring that do not make them sub-servient but which demonstrate that they have professional expertise. An historical examination of the ways in which these occupations have developed since the nineteenth century shows clearly that a major aspect has been the attempts to achieve professional status (Abbott and Wallace, Chapter 2 in this volume). These occupational strategies are themselves often based implicitly on a 'trait model' of what a profession is. Also an examination of the history of nursing and social work challenges a passive interpretation of women's subordination. Women have challenged male domination and developed strategies to achieve professional status and these have been resisted by men and by some women. Rather than rejecting the claim made to professional status by social work and nursing, it might be more relevant to recognise that this model of a profession is based upon man-made criteria in the first place. Maria Lorentzon (Chapter 5) argues that social work and nursing are female professions different from rather than inferior or subordinate to the male-dominated professions. However, not all aspects of professionalization can be reduced to gender alone. Phil Bean (Chapter 10) indicates that the conflict between the professional groups he describes is not so much a struggle between the sexes, as the resistance by psychiatrists to police making diagnoses of mental disorder.

Key elements in any claim to professional status seem to be autonomy or control over work, a clearly defined monopoly over an area of work and a knowledge base. It is in these areas that both social work and nursing have attempted to demonstrate that they are professions and in which they have also been challenged. Neither social workers or nurses have autonomous control as practitioners over their work. Not only are they closely supervised by their superiors in their day-to-day work, but (in the case of social work) even those who supervise them are frequently not qualified in their discipline (C. Davies, 1982). Nor do they necessarily have a monopoly over an area of work — caring work is often seen as women's work and closely identified with what women are supposed to be doing for their families without payment in any case. The Nurses Act 1918 established the General Nursing Council which supervises the training and examining of nurses — but the title 'nurse' is not reserved exclusively for those on the register of qualified nurses. The Central Council for the Education and Training of Social Work approves courses training social workers. However, no qualification is necessary to practice as a social worker and, as Roger Sibeon (Chapter 7) points out, recent moves to reform social work training (if implemented) could mean the removal of the distinction between social workers and social service workers. Nurses and social workers have also attempted to develop knowledge bases or theories that underpin their work — nursing theory and social work theory. Both borrow eclectically from the social sciences, but it is generally felt that neither occupation has yet developed an autonomous body of knowledge that is the basis of expert professional practice. Indeed, some have argued that nurses and social workers can do little more for clients than the well intentioned lay person. This claim is reinforced by the identification of their work as what women do 'naturally'. Thus, social workers and nurses have not, as yet, successfully claimed professional status — that is, they are not generally recognized as professions equal to other occupations such as medicine and law.

Nursing is seen as a traditional female role, and in the popular image at least, as subordinated to medical control. Nurses are seen as carrying out the instructions of doctors. The possibilities of nurses achieving professional status are limited as a consequence of its association in popular ideology with mundane bedside drudgery that is seen as 'women's work' (Gamarnikow, 1978). The characteristic features of nursing are low pay, low prestige, unsocial hours, high turnover and lack of job autonomy (see Lesley Mackay, Chapter 3 in this volume). The development of educational programmes for nurses has not superficially improved their status in the medical hierarchy either in the hospital or the community context (C. Davies, 1982).

Social work, similarly, has been associated with female roles. While it has not been dominated in the same way as nursing by other occupations in the division of labour, social workers have nevertheless not established themselves as autonomous practitioners. The moves towards an all qualified profession with a theoretical training undertaken in institutions of higher education went some way towards establishing the role of social workers, but this is now being challenged, with a case being made for more practical training (see Roger Sibeon, Chapter 7 in this volume). The status of social workers has been severely dented by the publicity given to cases where children under social work supervision have been battered to death by their parents, and cases where it is argued that social workers have broken up families unnecessarily by taking children into care. Whilst individual social workers may be accused of negligence or of acting over-zealously, these cases also give credence to the view that social workers have no 'specialist' expertise and should instead have more 'common sense'. Social workers are generally employed within bureaucratic organizations and are closely supervised in their work by managers — they are accountable to their employers (often local government) as well as their clients.

However, by focusing on debates about whether or not occupational groups including social workers and nurses are professionals we lose sight of other key qualities — and especially the power of occupational groups over clients. The power of these occupations tends to rest on their occupational positions, the legitimacy placed on them as a result of this and the power they exercise based on their claims to knowledge (see the articles by David McCallum and by Abbott and Sapsford, Chapters 8 and 9 in this volume). The caring professions are powerful because they not only aim to change and control behaviour, but also help to structure the context of social and cultural life in a more general sense — through their power to command definitions of reality by which the lives of their clients are shaped (see Abbott and Sapsford, Chapter 9). In other words, they create both the object of their intervention — the neglectful mother, the wayward teenager, the bad patient — and at the same time make these the targets of their intervention. Intervention is designed to normalize, to make subjects conform to the defined norms. In this model people are seen as having or being problems and the experts as having solutions — the knowledge to solve the problem. Nurses and social workers claim the right (power) to instruct, to tell people what they need to know and how they should act. To define someone as a client is to determine that they have a need and that the need can only be met by the expertise of the social worker or nurse. The professional, not the client, defines the problem, and the solution is seen to come out of the professional knowledge of the social worker or nurse.

Whilst sociologists have commonly drawn attention to the power exercised by social workers (although less so for nurses) and criticized them for being agents of social control, they have ignored two key interrelated factors: first, that clients of social workers tend to be predominantly female, and, second, that they are mainly working-class. Whilst the welfare state is partially an outcome of a history of struggles by the working class for better living conditions, it has also come to control them. Most social workers and nurses are female and they exercise control over women — much of the time working within patriarchal ideologies (Orr, 1986). The control they exercise is often designed to persuade clients to live their lives in ways they would not choose, rather than working with their clients to overcome their problems (A. Davies, 1987; Abbott and Sapsford, Chapter 9 in this volume).

We have argued that it is more profitable to examine what an occupational group does, what expertise its practitioners claim to have, how it intersects with other occupational groups in the division of labour and the strategies it adopts to improve its status *vis-à-vis* other groups, than merely to categorize occupations. In this way we can raise questions both about the relationships with their clients of those in client-centred occupations, the division of labour between occupations that share clients, and the strategies occupational groups use to maintain dominance over both clients and other occupations. In this respect it is important to note that social workers and nurses, in attempting to be upwardly mobile as professions, exclude and marginalize other groups: in the case of social workers, social service workers (see Roger Sibeon, Chapter 7 in this volume) and in the case of nurses the Enrolled and Auxiliary grades.

Social workers and nurses have used a variety of strategies to lay claim to the status of professional. 'Professional' in modern, capitalist societies is generally a term of approval and one that implies payment for special skills and proficiency. To claim to be a profession is to suggest independence, autonomy and control over work, but neither social workers nor nurses have achieved recognition as professional occupations, in terms of financial rewards or in terms of autonomy over work. Both groups have justified their strategies to achieve professional status by arguing that it would improve client/patient care. However, it is not clear that achieving professional status would necessarily do this. The strategies successfully used to achieve professional status by the medical profession seem to be as much about protecting and enhancing the status of doctors as protecting the public and providing a higher level of service. Jane Salvage (1985) has argued that if nursing became professionalized it would lead to nurses identifying with doctors rather than with ancillary and auxiliary staff, relatives and friends of the patients. This, she suggests, could strengthen barriers between nurses and patients and create barriers between workers, rather than encouraging them to work as a team to meet the needs of patients. She concludes by arguing that strategies to professionalize are less about meeting the needs of patients/clients, than about an occupational group pursuing its own narrow interests.

To conclude, we want to point to a key element, often ignored in sociological texts on the professions — the ways in which the words 'profession' and 'professionalism' are used in everyday language to *control* those who use or lay claim to the title. Social workers and nurses, as well as other professional and semi-professional groups, are often accused of 'acting un-professionally' — that is, of failing to put their patients or clients first (e.g. when they threaten industrial action in pursuit of higher wages or better conditions at work). To be 'professional', the caring professions are expected to be selfless, putting the needs of others before their own. In part this is not surprising, given that many of the workers in the semi-professions are female, and given the power of family ideology to define and circumscribe those occupations in the 'female sector' of the division of labour. Beyond this, however, another discourse comes in to play: the idea of profession-alism is used to police the actions of those who lay claim to a professional status — that is, certain standards of performance and behaviour are expected of them, standards set in essence from *outside* the control of the profession itself. Groups who aspire to professional status are laying themselves open to be controlled by externally defined standards — a 'pro-fessional discourse' which both defines what is to count as 'professional behaviour' and targets those who are perceived not to conform to it. The power of the discourse is used to control the behaviour of the aspiring pro-fession. One of the outcomes of this is that a sector of the middle class — including caring 'professionals' — are prepared, indeed in some cases eager, to accept the historical constraints of professional status in order to acquire what they see as its freedom of action. In turn, the discourse that defines pro-fessions has developed in tandem with *male* specialisms such as medicine and the law and incorporates a range of essentially patriarchal assumptions and definitions which then become incorporated into the new professions, whether or not they may be appropriate. Hence the idea of 'professionalism' serves contradictory functions in the case of the caring professions. On the one hand professionalism defines and enhances the nature of these occu-pational groups. On the other, given the uncertain nature of the knowledge bases to which they lay claim, it constrains the ways in which they are able to define their tasks and lays them open to attack on the grounds of structurally unprofessional conduct.

References

ABBOTT, P. A. and WALLACE, C. (1990) *An Introduction to Sociology: Feminist Perspectives*, London, Routledge.

DAVIES, A. (1987) 'Hazardous Lives — Social Work in the 1980s: A view from the left', in LONEY, M., BOCOCK, B., CLARKE, J., COCHRANE, A., GRAHAM, P., and WILSON, M. (Eds) *The State or the Market*, London, Sage.

DAVIES, C. (1982) 'The regulation of nursing: an historical comparison of Britain and the USA', in ROTH, J. (Ed.) *Research in the Sociology of Health Care*, 2, pp. 121–60.

ETZIONI, A. (1969) *The Semi-Professions and their Organisation*, New York, Free Press; London, Collier Macmillan.

FRIEDSON, E. (1986) *Professional Powers: A Study of the Institutionalisation of Formal Knowledge*, Chicago and London, University of Chicago Press.

GAMARNIKOW, E. (1978) 'Sexual division of labour: the case of nursing', in KUHN, A. and WOLPE, A. (Eds) *Feminism and Materialism*, London, Routledge.

ILLICH, I. *et al.* (1977) *Disabling Professions*, London, Boyars.

JOHNSON, T. (1972) *Professions and Power*, London, Macmillan.

MINFORD, P. (1987) 'The Role of the Social Sevices: a view from the New Right', in LONEY, M., BOCOCK, B., CLARKE, J., COCHRANE, A., GRAHAM, P. and WILSON, M. (Eds) *The State or the Market*, London, Sage.

ORR, J. (1986) 'Feminism and Health Visiting', in WEBB, C. (Ed.) *Feminist Practice in Women's Health Care*, Chichester, Wiley.

PARRY, N. and PARRY, J. (1976) *The Rise of the Medical Profession*, London: Croom Helm.

SALVAGE, J. (1985) *The Politics of Nursing*, London, Heinemann.

2
Social Work and Nursing: A History

Pamela Abbott and Claire Wallace

In this chapter we intend to examine the development of nursing and social work as caring professions. In doing so, we are presenting a *reading* of the processes and stereotypes involved in the transformation of nursing and social work from predominantly philanthropic work undertaken by unpaid ladies into modern occupational groups. Our argument is that there is no such thing as a 'factual' history, but rather, accounts or readings of history that are influenced by the theoretical position of the authors and the purpose for which the history is written. In our reading of the history of nursing and social work we are heavily influenced by feminist, Marxist and Foucauldian theories — the main approach being a Foucauldian one. In taking a Foucauldian approach we consider how nurses and social workers come to exercise power and regulate social life through the development of knowledge bases which are in turn embedded in discourses emerging at different points in time. The claim to these knowledge bases as 'truth' — as operating beyond everyday common sense — leads to the legitimating of particular spheres of professional expertise; and similarly the weakness or ambiguity in these knowledge claims can lead to the challenging of professional expertise. Consequently, it is important to look at the historical emergence of different discourses as they relate to the various caring professions and the way in which they were institutionalized through welfare bureaucracies. The Foucauldian approach differs from other approaches as it takes a non-essentialist view of these claims to knowledge or 'truth'. Thus, we can examine how discourses surrounding the idea of the family, crime, the nature of deviance, poverty and health emerged, the ways in which they structured the conceptual world and their effects on professional practice, without having to concern ourselves with their 'truth' or 'falsehood'.

Social Work

Social work developed out of a number of disparate voluntary, charitable and paid nineteenth-century endeavours associated with Victorian philanthropy. The Charities Organization Society, founded in London, is often seen as the main foundation of contemporary generic (local authority) social work. At the same time, the National Society for the Prevention of Cruelty to Children was established and its officers began to develop child protection work. Hospital almoners, the forerunners of medical (hospital) social workers were originally employed in the voluntary hospitals to determine which patients could afford to pay for treatment and which needed charity help. Along with probation officers, an occupation that developed from the court missionaries, they were amongst the first social work groups to develop formal training and a professional vocation. During the First World War both groups established professional associations. Residential social work developed out of the work of voluntary bodies such as Dr Barnardo's Waifs and Strays, the Church of England Children's Society and the National Children's Homes. These bodies were set up to care for abandoned and neglected children.

Social work developed to deal with various problem groups — groups such as the sick, the old, the poor, the workless and the criminal. In the nineteenth century there was a general fear of the 'dangerous' classes and it was thought that if left uncontrolled they would contaminate the respectable and healthy members of society. A response to this was the monitoring and surveillance of the lower-class groups in society, although the concept of institutionalization — the poor in the workhouse, the mentally ill in asylums — dominated nineteenth-century thinking about social problems (see, for example, Scull, 1977). This, however, was not a complete answer — it was attacked by some reformers, and in any case the majority of those perceived as 'problems' were not incarcerated. Many of the mentally ill and mentally handicapped were left to be 'cared' for by their families and some workhouse unions provided outdoor relief for able-bodied paupers. Increasingly, the view was taken that at least some of the 'problem' groups — the deserving poor — could be normalized; that is, they could become respectable self-supporting members of society if given the right kind of assistance and guidance. At the same time evangelical Christians with a strong religious commitment to charity began to argue that charity *per se* demoralized the poor. They argued that the deserving poor should be trained in thrift and self-help. They further suggested that the administration of the Poor Law needed to be tightened up so that it had the intended deterrent effect: that is, that the undeserving poor should *not* be given outdoor relief but should be admitted to the workhouse. Finally, they argued that there needed to be rationalization of private charity in order to find ways of coping with the 'clever' paupers — the paupers who abused the system and encouraged the corruption and demoralization of the 'honest poor'. The outcome of this was the founding of the Charities Organization Society (COS) in London in 1869. It was concerned to ensure that a clear distinction was drawn between the undeserving and the deserving poor. It was underpinned by moral values that were used to determine which individuals were 'in real need' and which were 'playing the system'. The dominant *laissez-faire* ideology that under-pinned its moral values saw two causes of poverty: those who were poor because of natural disasters (such as widowhood) and those who were poor due to their own 'moral failing' — that is, an unwillingness to work, or spending money on drink and gambling. It thus linked with an individual-istic explanation for the causes of poverty. The deserving poor, those whose poverty was no fault of their own and who displayed willingness to help themselves and exhibited the moral virtues of thrift, sobriety and self-disci-pline, were to be assisted. The 'clever' paupers, however, were to be admitted to the workhouse.

Social case work developed out of the work of the Charities Organiz-ation Society. The officers of this organization were concerned to assess and classify different kinds of applicants — and, therefore, different kinds of poverty — to ensure that the 'clever paupers' who were undeserving, did not take advantage of the system. The religious orientation of the organization meant that they were also concerned with moral regulation and inculcating habits of thrift, providence and industry in their clients. This concern was embodied in the 'case work' approach to individual applicants whereby their families were investigated and they were encouraged to conform to particular 'virtuous' middle-class models of what the family life of the poor should consist of in order to qualify. Those given assistance were followed up so that it could be seen how the money was spent and the officers kept 'case notes' for all those who were assisted. This case work approach also identified the family as a particular site of intervention, the place where social problems arose and where they could be prevented or overcome. The family was therefore a subject of moral regulation and surveillance in these instances (Clarke, 1988). However, in becoming this, the family was constituted in particular ways. First there was the separation of the public and private spheres, the family being located in the private sphere and its members being seen as 'naturally' subject to patriarchal authority; what a man did to his wife, or parents to their children, was their own concern, not that of the state. Furthermore it was seen as the responsibility of the father to control his family. For this reason, it was at first the concern of welfare organizations to ensure the proper conformity of family members to this model of the patri-archal nuclear family. However, by the end of the nineteenth century it was recognized that the individuals could also be abused by their own family members. Campaigns by the National Society for Prevention of Cruelty to Children (NSPCC) and Dr Barnardo's Children's Homes — assisted by the evolving ideology of childhood as a stage of individual development when people could be saved from vice by an improved environment — led to the intervention of welfare officers in the private sphere by taking children away from homes deemed to be unsuitable.

If patriarchal authority was the means for regulating the family, women were supposed to be the *moral* guides for the household. They had to be more temperate, more religious and more sexually pure than men and their main role in life was seen as serving others dutifully. The officers of the COS thus targeted mothers particularly, since they were seen as being responsible for improving the morals of their husbands and children. This image of Victorian femininity also provided a model for the women who ran the Charities Organization Society and for other welfare professions, as we shall see later.

An attempt to set up training for COS social workers was made through the initiation of a 'School for Sociology' in 1903 which was later incorporated into the London School of Economics in 1912. This development coincided with the decline of the COS view of poverty and the change to a more 'scientific' and professional model. Paid workers were employed by the COS and other voluntary societies to work alongside the volunteers and once a body of paid workers was established, they began to develop a career structure. As the century progressed, social workers accumulated more specialized functions — child care, adoption and fostering, the elderly, the mentally handicapped and so on. Each of these involved the further elabor-ation of classifications and theories of disadvantage and in doing so more secular models emerged. The decline of moral theories of poverty and the advent of trained and paid workers resulted in a demand for a systematic body of knowledge on which social work practice could be based — a basis for *professional* social work. The training that emerged had three key elements: social studies, the theory of case work and supervised practical experience. Of these, the theory of case work was the key to the theory and practice of social work, providing the foundation for social work theory. Psychology replaced religious morality as the 'science' which legitimated intervention and served to classify different forms of deprivation. Psychology argued for the existence of a set of developmental stages — childhood, adolescence, normal adulthood and old age — through which people passed and during which they had particular needs. The family was seen as central to 'normal' psycho-social development. Psychology prescribes the 'norms' of behaviour and this 'knowledge' became the basis of professional social work intervention in families. By defining the normal, psychology also defined the abnormal and this provided the knowledge for targeting individuals and families as objects of intervention. Childhood was a period of special care and nurture during which the child must not be allowed to fall into vicious ways, and old age was a period of dependency and decrepitude. Likewise, sociology stressed the social origins and context of particular social problems. However, psychology legitimated the role of individual case work, and the family as the site of intervention. Social workers learned about the normative models of family life (often derived from middle-class families) which enabled them to classify families according to whether they were 'deviant' or 'normal' — deviant families included all those without conventional male household heads or those from ethnic minorities or different class cultures which did not conform to the models of the normal family held by those who taught or practised social work.

In the period before World War II the dominant model was that of the 'problem' family — families which increased the numbers in the 'social problem' groups by passing on physical and mental deficiencies from one generation to the next. This model focused attention on children as victims of physical neglect and deprivation. The blame was usually placed upon the mother for failing to care adequately for her children (for an account of similar influences in health visiting see Abbott and Sapsford, Chapter 9 in this volume). Children came to provide the main justification for the entry of social workers into families and thus gave impetus for the imagery of the neglected child during the Second World War. The Report of the Committee on Care of Children, published in 1946, recommended a specialized social work service for children. The 1948 Children's Act established local authority children's departments which were to employ specialist trained social workers: child care officers responsible for working with families and children in need of care. These developments provided the foundations for the development of professional social work after World War II in Britain. At the same time, separate services were provided for the physically and mentally sick, the handicapped and the elderly. The child care officers appointed by the local authorities were the main group of qualified social workers existing at the end of the Second World War. Psychology continued to dominate the theory and practice of social work, and case work was likewise the main paradigm used.

However, the paradigm changed and the theories of Bowlby and others stressed the importance of maternal bonding and the problems associated with maternal deprivation and 'latchkey' children. As the child care services developed the trained workers began to advocate preventative work. Hence, the Children and Young Persons Act of 1963 provided children's departments with the power to give financial or other help to prevent the reception of children into care. The emphasis was on keeping families, particularly mothers and children, together. Social problems were blamed upon ignorance rather than poverty and the problem family characterized as lacking in social skills, so that the social worker should interpret their problems on their behalf and act as intermediary between them and the state. By the 1960s, poverty was not thought to be the main problem facing 'problem families'. Rather, it was their inability to cope with an increasingly complex society:

> The service that is needed must set out by concentrating on the few families that get into serious difficulties but would be available from the beginning to all those who wish to make use of it (it would be a 'family casework service', not a 'problem families service'). It must be manned by workers with a sensitive understanding of family relationships, and special skills in mobilising the will and the energy of the bewildered, anxious and aggressive people (thus it would be based primarily on the skilled use of personal relationships, rather then the provision of material help and expert advice) (Donnison and Stewart, 1958, p. 7).

However, it was not until the early 1970s, following the Seebohm Committee Report (1968), that state social work was reorganized into unified local authority departments charged with providing statutory and non-statutory services for those in need. This established the form that social work takes in Britain today — generic departments with generic social work training and methods based on psychological theories of interpersonal relations within the family. The child care workers exerted the strongest influence on the work of the new departments with their emphasis on case work, and the main focus of work is still seen as being with families and young children. Social workers were divided into two categories: field and residential. The former generally had a professional qualification validated by the Central Council for Education and Training in Social Work and awarded after study at an institution of higher education. The latter staff received less training and were less well qualified, being seen generally as social service staff rather than as professional social workers (see Roger Sibeon, Chapter 7 in this volume).

Although social work has developed from voluntary work based on moral values into an occupation consisting of paid workers basing their interventions on 'scientific' knowledge, it is not securely established as a profession and its areas of expertise remain vague and ill-defined. Over the last twenty years social work has been attacked by the left — for exercising social control and for failing to tackle the root causes of social problems — and by the right for being naive 'do-gooders' trying to take away people's sense of responsibility. Furthermore, successive scandals in child abuse have helped to vilify social workers in the papers, especially after the much-publicized deaths of Maria Colwell and Jasmine Beckford. Social workers are vilified for leaving 'at risk' children with their families as in these cases, and for un-justified interference or breaking up families, as in the much-publicized Cleveland scandal. This has led to a further crisis in confidence for a fragile profession. Cuts in welfare benefits, and the burgeoning numbers of social work clients with rising unemployment, rising numbers of elderly and the recent discovery of child sexual abuse, have meant that social workers are mainly concerned with responding to crises rather than preventing crises from occurring (if they ever did that) and their role has been one of rationing increasingly scarce resources (see the Barclay Committee Report, 1982).

These criticisms have led some to challenge the whole basis of social work professional practice; that is, to challenge the truth of the scientific discourses — mainly psychology — on which social workers base their practice. However, the various scandals have led to calls within the profession for more broadly based and extended training as the basis of professional expertise and the need for social workers to enter the profession as mature entrants with some experience of voluntary work — that is, the solution is seen as better training and better selection. There nevertheless exists a large penumbra of untrained and semi-trained volunteers who undertake much social service work and this would seem to undermine the claims of social work to professional expertise and knowledge, as does their apparent inability to carry out diagnostic and preventative work in the area of child abuse.

However, it is nonetheless essential to recognize the role that social workers do and can play in helping to protect the least powerful and most vulnerable members of society.

Nursing

The origins of nursing also lie in the nature of nineteenth-century philan-thropy and in discourses of the family. Whilst doctors and medical specialists amongst the plethora of other professional paid healers were known from the Middle Ages, their activities were fairly narrowly defined, and many people could not afford to see them. Much healing work was undertaken by women and was seen as part of their domestic routine. By the nineteenth century, however, allopathic medicine had successfully come to claim a monopoly of medical expertise and in Britain this was given state recognition in the 1852 Medical Act which gave medical doctors monopolistic rights (see Stacey, 1989). Independent nurses and midwives continued to practise but were condemned by social reformers such as Florence Nightingale for being inexpert, unprofessional and uninformed by recent medical theories. However, we have to remember that Nightingale was keen to promote an alternative, more formal kind of professional intervention.

In the late nineteenth century, at the same time as modern scientific medicine was gaining its hegemonic position and female health workers were being condemned by reformers, there emerged a concern for the health of the poor and with public health generally. This took the form of efforts to prevent the spread of epidemics such as cholera and a concern with eugenics — breeding the right sort of people fit to rule, work and fight for the Empire. In the early twentieth century, these concerns were highlighted by the poor standard of health of recruits to the Boer War and later the First World War prompting a series of reforms to improve the nation's health. Linked to this was the fact that physical decay was associated with moral decay. The family and particularly mothers were made responsible for the health of other family members, as childhood became identified as a period of special personal growth when the individual needed protection from contamination and vice. Consequently mothers were discouraged from working, encouraged to be dependent upon male breadwinners and to be responsible for family health. Abbott and Sapsford (see Chapter 9) have demonstrated how health visitors were used to 'police' poor families and educate working-class mothers in these hygienic pursuits. It is evident from this that medical and moral discourses were aligned. Nursing was established as a profession supplementary to medicine (Gamarnikow, 1978) but also heavily influenced by the hygiene discourse.

Nursing emerged in the late nineteenth century as a distinct occupational category in a form recognizable today. However, it is important to recognize that the origins of contemporary nursing are diverse and are reflected in the nursing specialisms that exist today — adult nursing, children's nursing, mental health nursing, mental handicap nursing, midwifery and community nursing (health visiting and district nursing). In the rest of this chapter we are going to look in detail at two types of nursing: first, adult nursing, which exemplifies the development of an occupational group to meet the medical needs of doctors as medical practice changed through the late eighteenth and nineteenth centuries; second, midwifery as an example of an occupation that became subordinated to medicine in the process of medical men striving to achieve a dominant role in the medical division of labour.

Hearn (1982) has argued that the process of professionalization is a process of male assumption of control over female tasks. Thus as male doctors acquire the status of a profession they not only exclude female healers from practising but gain control over female workers, who take on a subordinate role in the medical division of labour.

Midwives

Women healers retained control over childbirth for a much longer period than they did over healing generally, but even in midwifery they began from the 1660s to have their dominant role challenged by male midwives (obstetricians), the latter claiming to have scientific knowledge and technical expertise not possessed by female midwives. It is possible that the origins of male midwifery relate to the invention of the obstetrics forceps, or more simply that it was just another example of males attempting to take over a field previously dominated by females. However, there was opposition to male midwifery firstly from the general public (who thought it was indecent), secondly from female midwives (on account of the threat to their livelihood) and finally from established medical men (who saw this as degrading women's work and not part of medicine at all).

It is not evident why male midwives were gradually able to usurp the role of the female midwives. Although the invention of obstetric forceps was certainly a breakthrough and their use was restricted to members of the guild of barber-surgeons from which women were excluded, the number of cases where they helped was small and the risk of infection and death as a result of their use was enormous. Women were also excluded from practising in the lying-in hospitals, but these hospitals only took in low risk cases and risk of infection and death was much higher than for home delivery. Probably the key factor was the claim of medical men to have access to scientific (and therefore true) knowledge which female midwives lacked, and the way support was given for this claim by the trend for wealthy people to employ male midwives from the seventeenth century onwards.

However, it was not until the late nineteenth century that medical doctors accepted that midwifery should be undertaken and controlled by men. During the nineteenth century the Colleges of Physicians and Surgeons both argued against doctors' involvement in midwifery, but by 1850 lectures in midwifery were being given in British medical schools and by 1866 proficiency in it was necessary for qualification as a medical practitioner. The claim by doctors to control childbirth was made on a basis that medical men had superior knowledge, a claim that had been generally accepted as medical men successfully excluded or marginalized other forms of healing and other practitioners:

> By 1880 a great advance had been made in the science and art of midwifery. This was due chiefly to the introduction of male practitioners, many of whom were men of learning and devoted to anatomy, the groundwork of obstetrics (Spicer, 1927, quoted in Oakley, 1980, p. 11).

This claim was not justified on medical grounds. In the nineteenth century a quarter of all women giving birth in hospital died of puerperal fever, and those delivered at home were more likely to be infected if they were attended by a male doctor rather than a female midwife. Puerperal fever was particularly a risk from male doctors because they moved between the sick, the dead and parturient women. Nevertheless, medical men were determined to gain control of midwifery and to determine the role of female midwives — to establish a division of labour between them and the female midwives. Thus they set out to demarcate what areas were rightfully theirs at the same time as defending medical prerogative. The struggle between medical men and female midwives since the seventeenth century had begun to establish a distinction between assistance at childbirth and intervention in childbirth — a distinction between 'normal' and 'abnormal' childbirth. Only male doctors (qualified medical practitioners) were allowed to use forceps and to intervene surgically. The Midwifery Registration Act of 1902 resulted in the registration and education of midwives coming under the control of medical men, and a doctor had to be called if anything went wrong with a delivery. A major reason why doctors did not usurp the role of midwives was that they realized that there was no way in which they could meet the demand — in the late nineteenth century seven out of every nine births were attended by female midwives. Also, many doctors did not want to attend poor women. Doctors thus deskilled and deprofessionalized midwives, and while female midwives continued to attend poor women in childbirth, doctors attended the wealthy. Medical domination of childbirth continues in the late twentieth century, and indeed it could be argued that it has increased because the majority of births take place in hospital under the (official) control of a consultant, and because of the increased use of medical terminology. Whilst most women are actually delivered by a (female) midwife, the ultimate control remains in the hands of the (generally male) obstetrician. The consequence of this is that midwives are not seen as playing a different role to doctors but as being subordinate to doctors. In order to free themselves from this control and establish themselves as an autonomous profession they not only have to challenge the need for medical supervision of their work, but establish that theirs is a particular kind of work, distinct from medical work, and that they have a unique knowledge and expertise which underlies their practice. The medicalization of childbirth has not only brought women under the control of medical men, but also denied an autonomous area of work for midwifery — midwives are now seen to work with medical knowledge, rather than with a distinct body of knowledge over which they have exclusive rights.

Adult Nursing

Nurses, too, play a subordinate role in the medical division of labour. Nursing has always been and continues to be a predominantly female province. Most nursing is of course done by women as unpaid carers in the domestic sphere; this has been, and still is, a major barrier to nurses arguing that they have specialized knowledge and expertise necessitating a long theoretical as well as practical training and justifying a claim to professional status. However, nursing in the public sphere is also a predominantly female occupation. Whilst caring for the sick was undertaken in a variety of institutions in the past, it was not until the middle of the nineteenth century that nursing emerged as a separate occupation. Prior to that, nursing in voluntary hospitals was seen as a form of domestic work that required little specific training, and was usually undertaken by married women doing little different for their patients than they did for their families at home. The demarcation between nurses and patients was blurred — the able-bodied convalescent patients were expected to help the nurses with the domestic work on the wards. Paid helpers were also employed in private households to assist with nursing the sick. The poor would have used handywomen who often acted as midwives while the better off would have employed private nurses who might or might not have had some experience of hospital nursing.

The reform of the nursing profession is often attributed to Florence Nightingale who claimed that nursing was done mainly at home by those 'who were too old, too weak, too drunken, too dirty, too sordid or too bad to do anything else' (quoted in Abel-Smith, 1960, p. 53). The argument that nurses needed training, and the recognition by doctors that bedside medicine meant that patients needed monitoring, developed before Florence Nightingale's reforms. From the 1830s doctors had begun to develop new ways of practising medicine and to argue that they needed a new type of assistant who could monitor the patients. At the same time the sister model (based on the model of religious orders) began to develop in the voluntary hospitals — working-class women did the nursing work and were supervised by middle-class women using household managerial skills which they had learned from supervising servants. Many of the sisters were motivated by religion, undertaking nursing as a calling — a vocation. However, Florence Nightingale did attempt to develop nursing as an occupation and to recruit middle-class women who would receive training — a training based on organized experience. These reforms took place in the voluntary hospitals and from that time it began to be argued that workhouse infirmaries should employ skilled nurses rather than use pauper women. The model developed in both the voluntary and the poor law hospitals of a small number of trained nurses (sisters) supervising the work of trainees and untrained staff.

While Florence Nightingale recognized the need for trained nurses, she trained them in obedience, so that in the division of labour between nurses and doctors, nurses were seen and saw themselves as subordinates of the doctors and as under medical control. Furthermore, she stressed that nursing was a vocation, not a profession, and accepted the prevailing ideas of a nursing hierarchy with a stress on strict obedience and control over moral behaviour both in and out of work. Both nurses and probationers were expected to 'live in' at the hospital, were strictly controlled in their behaviour both at work and during non-working hours and had no set hours of work, emphasizing the cloistered separateness of the nursing community. This model was reinforced by the idea of a vocation — a calling: the selfless sacrifice of the nurse to the needs of the patient. Nor did Nightingale challenge the link between womanhood and nursing. Gamarnikow (1978) has pointed out that in the Nightingale model, nurses were still responsible for the cleaning of wards as well as the care of patients. She suggests that the relationship between doctor and nurse paralleled the relationship between the Victorian husband and the wife in the family. The nurse looked after the physical and emotional environment, while he, the doctor, decided what the really important work was and how it should be done. Thus the good nurse was the good mother, concerned with caring for her patients. This reflected Victorian models of dutiful femininity and the family already described. Because nursing was a female profession its characteristics of duty and sub-servience were stressed rather than status or rewards. The subservience of nurses to doctors was given 'scientific' legitimacy because of the basis of nursing knowledge. Nursing did not develop an autonomous body of knowledge but the nursing tasks emerged out of the 'sanitary idea' and this gave coherence to the disparate tasks undertaken by nurses — medical tasks delegated by doctors, plus care for the patient's physical needs and the maintenance of the cleanliness of the wards (C. Davies, 1976). As a consequence of this the only role left available for the trained nurse was not that of autonomous practitioner but the management of trainee nurses and untrained helpers.

In the twentieth century, whilst nurses no longer see themselves as handmaidens of doctors, they have remained trapped in their status as subordinate to doctors. In 1918 the Nursing Register was introduced, and the Nurses Act 1943 established the lower grade of State Enrolled Nurses as well as State Registered Nurses, but neither kind were recognized as independent practitioners. Ann Williams (1987) has argued that the subordinate role of nurses is exemplified in the ways drugs are administered in hospitals:

> . . . doctors prescribe drugs and nurses administer drugs. Here is
> an example of nurses as 'handmaidens' to doctors. They have no
> say in prescribing drugs. They are not authorised to prescribe what
> they give. Yet they are accountable for what they give, how much
> etc., etc. (Williams, 1987, p. 107).

The main struggle in the twentieth century has been between those who want nursing to become an autonomous profession and those who see nursing as more of a vocation and are more concerned with practice than with developing theories to underpin practice. This struggle started in the nineteenth century between the professionals led by Mrs Fenwick and the vocationalists led by Florence Nightingale. The Nurses Registration Act of 1919 was a compromise between these groups. It resulted in the establishment of a register of trained nurses and the establishment of the General Nursing Council in 1920 which was charged in 1923 with maintaining a register and determining the conditions of entry to that register — that is, what examinations had to be passed in order to be placed on the register. Only nurses on the register could call themselves State Registered. However, whilst the 'registered nurse' title was protected this was *not* a prerequisite for employment as a nurse. The Act did not give nurses the power to control entry to the profession nor to oversee training, nor the monopoly of practice that, for example, the 1852 Medical Act had given medical doctors.

Nurses had not made a move towards a particular role nor had they gained autonomous control over their work. The outcome of this was that nursing continued to be an occupation that was based on a predominantly practical training and where the qualified supervised the unqualified trainees. The situation has not fundamentally changed since for either hospital or community nurses. Indeed it could be argued that subsequent changes have removed the managerial role of nurses rather than enabling them to gain fundamental autonomy and a particular role. The Salmon Report (1966) reflected the views of the nursing elite that trained nurses should predominantly be concerned with managerial and clinical aspects of nursing work and that routine 'dirty' work should be done by other groups under their control — state enrolled nurses, trainees and auxiliaries. This would enable the establishment of a career (managerial) status for nurses. This was based on an industrial model of line management and of professional managers. Emphasizing managerial aspects of promoted posts and the need for specific managerial skills as criteria for promotion has downgraded the need for the caring (female) qualities for nursing. In their search for a career ladder and higher status, nurses adopted a managerial solution that resulted in the tighter control of nursing staff and mitigated against the development of nurses as autonomous practitioners. Indeed it continued and developed the process by which most nursing work is done by the untrained and the trainee. Furthermore, the changes in management hierarchies in the 1980s following the Griffiths inquiry mean that nurses can now be managed by men nurses.

The fight between the managerialist faction and the professionalists has, however, continued. Those who emphasize a professional model for nursing have tended to be concentrated in the schools of nursing and advocate a more theoretical training for nursing and the development of nursing theory. This view influenced the Briggs Report (1972) and more recently the proposals for the Project 2000 which are in the process of being implemented. Whilst the Nurses, Midwives and Health Visitors Act of 1979 did not reflect the aspirations of the professionalists it is possible that Project 2000 may prove to do so, providing it allows for trainees to be supernumerary for most of their training and to have their qualifications validated by institutions of higher education. There will be an increased emphasis on theory as the basis of nursing practice. Grades of nursing (State Enrolled Nurse and Auxiliary Nurse) other than Registered Nurse will be abolished and a new assistant grade introduced but without the title 'nurse'.

However, a number of factors mitigate against the new Project 2000 nurse gaining professional status. It is unclear what the 'new' nurse will do that is different from existing qualified nurses — that is, managing the work of non-qualified nurses. The tight managerial structure of nursing has not been modified. Furthermore, developments such as the nursing process, which is seen as the basis for autonomous nursing work, will enable both qualified (supervisory) nurses and those whose work they are directing to be more strictly monitored and evaluated. Additionally, as the research of Kath Melia (1987) demonstrates, staff numbers make the implementation of the nursing process problematic and ward culture continues to emphasize 'getting the job done' and the routinization of nursing tasks rather than the diagnostic care, planning and implementation approach of the nursing process. Nursing, like social work, has not developed its own body of knowledge that provides the theoretical basis for practice and the syllabus for Nursing 2000 may reduce the control over nurse education or nurse educators as psychologists, sociologists and biologists from the collaborative institutions of higher education become involved in the planning and delivery of nurse education. It seems unlikely that doctors will, on the basis of Project 2000 training, come to see nurses as equal but different in the health care division of labour and it is more likely that they will continue to see nurses as inferior to medical practitioners. Nor are patients going to change their view of nurses as doctor's aides. Patients value what nurses do for them but they are unlikely to accord them the status of knowledgeable expert that they accord to doctors. The lack of power of nurses can be seen to be related to their inability to develop an autonomous knowledge base, to underpin an area of work where they are perceived as experts. (The one potential exception to this is health visiting — see Abbott and Sapsford, Chapter 9.) Nurses have failed to gain the necessary autonomy, prestige or power accorded to the status of professional.

Nursing in the late twentieth century is seen as a predominantly low paid female occupation, but there are clear ethnic and class divisions in nursing. The three grades of nursing — auxiliaries, state enrolled and state registered — form a clear hierarchy with little or no possibility of training to move up the qualification hierarchy. Women from ethnic minorities are concentrated in the auxiliary and state enrolled grades, and white middle-class women in the registered grade in the prestigious teaching hospitals. Furthermore, more men are entering nursing, and the new managerial structures introduced in the 1970s have resulted in a disproportionately large number of men appointed to management posts. Although men have been able to become general nurses only since 1943, they have increasingly moved into senior posts in what was once, as far as the nursing of physical illness was concerned, an all-woman and woman-managed occupation.

More recently, the reorganization of nursing suggested by the Griffiths Report (1983) and Project 2000 has emphasized the role of managerial control through financial constraints and the breaking down of nursing tasks. Griffiths himself was imported from Sainsbury's, a highly successful private retail company, to provide new models and ideas in public service.

Problems of Professionalization

It is evident from the discussion above that ideologies of deviance, the family and individual development are held in common by the caring professions. These professions are relatively recent and all have their roots in voluntary philanthropic work in the nineteenth century. But what does 'professional knowledge' consist of in these instances? First, an area of social life is defined as problematical and 'theories' about it emerge; secondly, caring professionals are familiar with the processes of administration within the welfare state through which that problem is managed and controlled. This is informed by various kinds of knowledge in which the professional is trained. Psychology has been particularly successful in establishing itself as a knowledge base because the positivistic background of the discipline lends itself to claims for scientific 'truth'. In addition the British Psychological Society — under pressure from clinical psychologists anxious to establish their professional base within the health service — has been concerned to erect professional barriers. In the past the BPS has defined which psychology degrees provide the necessary education for membership of the British Psychological Society. More recently, however, the BPS tried unsuccessfully to get the title 'psychologist' restricted to those with a recognized degree. They did manage to get an Act of Parliament restricting the use of the term Chartered Psychologist to those on the BPS register. Sociology has not attempted to do this since most sociologists would reject professional claims to positivistic knowledge and because the growth of sociology in Britain has been far more recent and more amorphous than that of psychology. Nevertheless, sociology is used in the training of all the caring professionals that we have identified here and its use is increasing rather than decreasing. Furthermore, particular specialisms within sociology — in health and illness or in crime — are identified with particular caring professions, although the theories and ideas which emerge are often critical rather than supportive of those professions. Furthermore the individualistic nature of intervention means sociological theories with an emphasis on structural explanations of social problems are seen as less relevant in day-to-day practice, although a more 'community work' approach to both social work and nursing is influenced by these more structural theories (see Ann Davies, 1987; Jean Orr, 1986).

Gender ideologies are an important factor in all the caring professions. First of all the idea of 'care' itself and the growth of this work from women's activities means that it is seen as an extension of female roles and therefore less privileged in status. Secondly, the clients, too, are often women and the caring professions impose certain gender ideologies upon them. Thus in the criminal justice system those in need of 'care protection and control' often from some unspecified sexual danger are more likely to be girls (Shacklady Smith, 1978). In social work, the professionals impose norms of motherhood and gender division of labour upon their clients in terms of their view of a 'normal' family. In nursing, midwifery and health visiting, women clients are expected to demonstrate adherence to social norms of femininity in order to exhibit correct health attitudes. Thirdly, many of the workers within those professions are women. Nursing is an almost exclusively female profession and constituted in the most obviously feminine way. However, many social workers, too, are women, especially those in basic rather than managerial grades. When professions become feminized they tend to suffer a lowering of rewards, prestige and status as has been well documented in the case of clerical workers. However, we can look at this another way, too, inasmuch as we can consider how male professionals came to claim so much 'caring' ground from women non-professionals, and in this way we can see professionalism as the means by which men are able to obtain better labour market positions for themselves. Another factor, perhaps, is that the clients of male professionals are normally rich and can pay for services they choose, whereas those of the caring professions are generally poor, have no choice as to what services they should receive and often resent the imposition of services and surveillance. In this way 'care' becomes merged into 'control' as the caring professions carry out statutory functions on behalf of the state.

All the professions have been affected by the last ten years of government by the New Right. The Thatcher government has been antagonistic towards professionals and has attacked their basis of power where possible either by removing their monopoly — as in the legal profession — or by financial controls — as in the medical profession. For those employed by the state there is also the possibility of lowering rewards directly and decreasing professional autonomy by increasing managerial control — as in the introduction of the national curriculum and new conditions of service for teachers. In addition, the use of managerial models of control and financial constraints imported from private industry would appear to be antithetical towards professional autonomy. However, the process has been contradictory. During the same period there has been a demand for the extension of training of caring professionals, and comprehensive plans for reorganization such as that introduced for social work and nursing will lead to the increased division of labour in those services between the qualified and the unqualified.

To conclude, it is evident that the development of the caring professions of social work and nursing since the nineteenth century have a lot in common with other welfare occupations such as teaching and probation work. However, the way in which 'caring' has come to be understood and its implications for professional status today need to be seen in terms of the historical development of ideologies surrounding it and its position in the social division of labour more generally.

References

ABBOTT, P. A. and SAPSFORD, R. J. (1988) 'The Body Politic: Health, Family and Society', Unit 11 of Open University Course D211 *Social Problems and Social Welfare*, Milton Keynes, Open University.
ABEL-SMITH, B. (1960) *A History of the Nursing Profession*, London, Heinemann.
BARCLAY REPORT (1982) *Social Workers: Their Role and Tasks*, London, Bedford Square Press.
BOWLBY, J. (1954) *Child Care and the Growth of Love*, Harmondsworth, Penguin.
BRIGGS REPORT (1972) *Report of the Committee on Nursing*, London, HMSO.
CLARKE, J. (1988) 'Social Work: the personal and the political', Unit 13 of Open University Course D211 *Social Problems and Social Welfare*, Milton Keynes, Open University.
DAVIES, A. (1987) 'Hazardous Lives — Social Work in the 1980's. A view from the left', in LONEY, M., BOCOCK, B., CLARKE, J., COCHRANE, A., GRAHAM, P. and WILSON, M. (Eds) *The State or the Market?* London, Sage.
DAVIES, C. (1976) 'Experience of Dependency and Control in Work: the case of nurses', *Journal of Advanced Nursing Studies*, 1, pp. 273–81.
DAVIES, C. (1982) 'The regulation of nursing: an historical comparison of Britain and the USA' in ROTH, J. (Ed.) *Research in the Sociology of Health Care*, 2, pp. 121–60.
DINGWALL, R. and LEWIS, P. (Eds) (1983) *The Sociology of the Professions*, London, Macmillan.
DONNISON, D. and STEWART, M. (1958) *The Child and the Social Sevices*, Fabian Pamphlet, London, Fabian Society.
GAMARNIKOW, E. (1978) 'Sexual division of labour: The case of nursing', in KUHN, A. and WOLPE, A. (Eds) *Feminism and Materialism*, London, Routledge.
GRIFFITHS REPORT (1983) *NHS Inquiry Report*, House of Commons Social Services Committee.
HEARN, J. (1982) 'Notes on Patriarchy, Professionalism and the Semi-professionals', *Sociology*, 16, 184–202.
MELIA, K. (1987) *Learning and Working: The Occupational Socialisation of Nurses*, London, Tavistock.
OAKLEY, A. (1980) *Subject Women*, London, Fontana.
OAKLEY, A. (1984) 'The Importance of Being a Nurse', *Nursing Times*, 12 December, pp. 24–7.
ORR, J. (1986) 'Feminism and Health Visiting', in WEBB, C. (Ed.) *Feminist Practice in Women's Health Care*, Chichester, Wiley.
RUESCHMEYER, D. (1973) *Lawyers and the Legal Society. A Comparative Study of the Legal Profession in Germany and the United States*, Cambridge, Mass., Harvard University Press.
SALMON REPORT (1966) *Report of the Committee on Senior Nursing Staff Structure*, London, HMSO.

SCULL, A. T. (1977) *Decarceration. Community Treatment and the Deviant. A radical view*, Englewood Cliffs, Prentice Hall.

SEEBOHM COMMITTEE (1968) *Report of the Committee on Local Authority and Allied Personal Social Services*, Cmnd. 3703, London, HMSO.

SHAKLADY SMITH, L. (1978) 'Sexist assumptions and female delinquency', in SMART, C. and SMART, B. (Eds) *Women, Sexuality and Social Control*, London, Routledge and Kegan Paul.

STACEY, M. (1989) *A Sociology of Health and Healing*, London, Unwin Hyman.

WILLIAMS, A. (1987) 'Making sense of feminist contributions to women's health', in ORR, J. (Ed.) *Women's Health in the Community*, Chichester, Wiley.

3
Nursing: Just Another Job?

Lesley Mackay

Attracting and keeping a nursing workforce has been, and will continue to be, a major concern for health service managers. Research into some of the issues relating to 'nurse recruitment and wastage' in a health authority in the North of England led us (Keith Soothill and myself) to ask some fundamental questions about nursing. Initial investigation of nurse recruitment and wastage demonstrated that the 'problem' was not why nurses left, but why, given the often appalling conditions under which they work, they stayed. The health authority's 'problem' was nurses' 'solution' to difficult and demanding work environments. As the research progressed, the original brief was broadened and other questions presented themselves: not only why nurses left, but why they did not leave; why did they stay; what did they get out of their work; what changes would encourage them to stay or persuade them to leave nursing. It soon became obvious that explanations would not simply be sought in individual differences, such as in particular satisfactions and dissatisfactions with work, but had to be situated within the systems in which nurses participate. Thus, we became concerned with the ideologies embedded in everyday working practices; professionalization; issues of gender; the systems of training and control, and many others.

Hopefully, our empirical work will be of use to those who develop and refine theories. Too often there is a search for spurious academic credibility by those undertaking empirical work: they 'tack on' aspects of this or that theory, or make it up as they go along. We were concerned with an 'unwrapping' of nurses' situation rather than with testing a specific theory. Obviously the questions we posed were informed by theory but we did not artificially limit ourselves by subscribing to any particular one. The place of theory is to inform the practice: in the way that the research is conducted; the methods which are used; in the selection of aspects to investigate and in the comments and recommendations made. The use of theory should be eclectic and not arbitrarily narrow the focus of enquiry.

In looking at 'wastage' amongst nurses we found that movement by nurses from one job to another is both necessary and expected within the system. Indeed, for many nurses, staying only a short time in one place is seen as normal. A nurse's qualifications can act as a very useful passport to foreign parts. (For women who recognize the limitations placed on their activities in other jobs, this ability to be employed, and in great demand, overseas, may be a potent initial attraction.) For a nurse to stay on one ward for many years can be a sign of stagnation or a lack of ability to move elsewhere or achieve promotion. In order to achieve promotion, nurses usually have to undertake further training. Nurses who wish to train further often have to move to another health authority which offers the specific course they want. In order to obtain sufficient experience before putting herself forward for further training, a nurse may have to work in a variety of different specialties. For nurses, therefore, movement is regarded as natural. The need for movement is built into the system. The management in the health authority was in effect, although they didn't recognize it, complaining about the system in which nurses operate. (The concern expressed in the late 1970s was that nurses would remain too long in one post and there would not be enough movement. This was a 'problem' which had to be monitored — see Redfern (1978).) Movement, however, can be interpreted as providing corroboration to the view that nurses, as women, are less than serious in pursuing a career. Thus, they can be seen as flitting like butterflies from one job to another, from one hospital to another, and even from one country to another. (It is worth remembering that junior members of the medical profession are similarly required to keep moving.)

The 'problem' of nurse recruitment which management was facing in the 1980s was essentially a demographic one: a shrinking number of young people with the qualifications or interest to enter nursing. Nurses, it appeared, had been treated as a disposable workforce, because they were young, female and easily replaced. Evidence in support of this 'disposable workforce' explanation emerged from many different areas. The substantial demand for further training was largely unmet. Similarly, promotion and career opportunities had not been developed to meet the aspirations of nurses. There is a dearth of childcare facilities and the demand for flexible working hours was essentially unheeded. Needless to say, at a national level, demands for substantial increases in pay had been ignored. In the management of nurses, both in the area of training and service provision, assumptions appear to be made regarding nurses: they are only a short-term workforce, with little interest in promotion or career; they only wish to work until they have children; thereafter they will stay happily at home caring for their families. It is a misogynistic and limiting view of women.

These assumptions fit uneasily with the idea of vocation which a number of nurses hold regarding their work. The frequent mention of vocation led us to investigate nurses' orientations to work. We did this in two ways: firstly through a questionnaire study of 154 nurses who had left, and 435 nurses who were still working in a health authority in the North of England. Secondly, information about nurses' views on their work was obtained through in-depth semi-structured interviews with 50 'leavers' and 50 'stayers'.

Brian Francis of the Centre of Applied Statistics at Lancaster University undertook an analysis of the questionnaire data. Having used a 'cluster analysis' he developed a four category grouping of nurses and their attitudes to their work. Using attitudinal questions such as 'What improvements are necessary to encourage trained nurses to stay?' and 'Does nursing offer sufficient career opportunities?', Brian Francis built up a picture of nurses' views of their jobs.

The first group was identified as seeing nursing as a vocation (18 per cent) — the problems reported by others in nursing were least evident to this group. Whatever the trials and tribulations of the job, they would continue to nurse. Two further groups of nurses saw nursing in terms of a career. The first group (18 per cent) of career orientated women sought a well-paid career whether in nursing or elsewhere. For the others who wanted a career (19 per cent), they were interested primarily in a career in nursing. They were committed to nursing and intended to 'battle it out' in the NHS. Nurses in this group would be unlikely to sacrifice their careers for their children. And it was from this group that there was the greatest demand for improvements regarding childcare facilities. The fourth group (28 per cent) of nurses saw nursing simply as a job. (Seventeen per cent of the nurses were not included in any of these groups.) Nurses, predictably, are not a homogeneous group.

The largest single group see nursing simply as just another job. They do not feel particularly attached to nursing and might leave if and when the opportunity arises. (Given the failure by the health service to meet the demands of so many nurses, it is perhaps surprising that the proportion of nurses in the group is not larger.) This group tended also to be family-centred and less concerned with a career. For these, as nursing is just a job, pay needs to be good. Many nurses in this group indicated they would be attracted by the private sector in health care.

Among these attitudes to work, the belief that nursing is a vocation is particularly significant. It is this notion of having, or the need for, a vocation which distinguishes nursing from most other occupations. Although not all nurses, by any means, subscribe to the belief that having a vocation for nursing is necessary, the idea of vocation is embedded in many of the accepted practices and attitudes within nursing. The dictionary definition (Concise Oxford Dictionary) of vocation is 'a divine call to, sense of fitness for, a career or occupation'. A vocation is commonly associated with those who enter the ministry or a religious order. It is no coincidence that both nuns and nurses use the title of sister: calling up the notion of familial and non-sexual love. (There is a notable overlap and common interest between nuns and nurses in the hospice movement.) In everyday activities, vocation is linked with being of service to others and putting others before oneself. Thus can nurses be called 'dedicated' and 'angels'. (It is worth noting that no other members of the modern health care team take recourse to the notion of vocation. Rather, the need for technical skill and expertise is emphasized while the personal characteristics and orientations of the radiographer, doctor, occupational therapist, etc., go largely unremarked.)

The way in which the idea of vocation is entrenched in nursing stems from the nineteenth century. It owes a great deal to Florence Nightingale's perception of what constitutes a 'good nurse'. She laid emphasis on character: on nurses being devoted and selfless. At the same time great emphasis was laid on the need for discipline. In the latter part of the nineteenth century there was a heated and lengthy debate regarding whether or not nurses should be registered. Nightingale (surreptitiously) opposed registration. The pro-registration argument emphasized the need for skill and training and sought professional status for nursing. The tension between these two opposing views of nursing is still apparent today.

The findings of Brian Francis regarding the relatively small number of nurses who are classified as seeing nursing as a vocation should not obscure the insidious and substantial effects of the ideology within nursing. Although nurses may not identify *themselves* as having a vocation, they may nevertheless subscribe to, or accept, some of the unspoken assumptions related to vocation in nursing. The majority of nurses say that it is the patients who make the job. Nurses say they like helping and looking after people. They are aware that they are doing a job which others will not or could not do. It is the awareness that special qualities are needed in nursing which distinguishes it from other jobs. The wish to be of service together with the need for special qualities act to reinforce the belief that nurses need to have a vocation.

The ramifications for nurses in accepting the idea of vocation are extensive. For example, in the questionnaire survey it became apparent that pay was a cause of considerable dissatisfaction. However, during the course of the interviews nurses' complaints of pay were seldom made regarding themselves but in respect of colleagues: nursing assistants, learners, enrolled nurses, etc. Accepting the notion of vocation leads to the 'I-will-always-manage' sentiment which in turn resulted in less anger about tangible benefits than might be expected in other occupations. It also helps explain the remarkably low salary levels in nursing. Thus, by holding to a notion of vocation, nurses' demands for more pay are muted. In turn, demands for higher salary levels are presented by nurses as simply wanting enough to live on, not for luxuries or other self-indulgences.

Having a vocation affects the nature of trade union membership and activity. Unable to put oneself first means that one doesn't complain, particularly through 'self-seeking' organizations such as trade unions. Nurses tend to join professional associations and seek improvements in their employment conditions quietly. Attitudes to trade unions are often lukewarm. Similarly, most nurses would not go on strike — although there is an increasing anger regarding what is seen as the mistreatment of nurses' goodwill by recent governments. Increasingly vociferous demands for improvements in conditions and a greater willingness to take some form of action (working to rule or striking) are becoming evident. Partly the anger being expressed is on behalf of patients, but many nurses are now angry on their own behalf as well. Yet nurses do not give full expression to their anger. This seems to be due to a seldom voiced belief amongst nurses that because they eschew speaking out for themselves, others must speak out for them. It sounds rather like being unable to ask for the salt at the dinner table in the nunnery and having to wait until another offers it to you.

Existing alongside the idea of vocation is a belief that nursing should establish itself as a profession. By following this path, it is argued that nursing would be accorded greater respect by other members of the health care team, particularly by the medical profession. At the same time, nurses would be in a stronger position to demand a salary that reflected the responsibility and commitment required from nurses. Curiously, the effect on nurses' actions of having a professional or a vocational perspective on nursing may be the same. Neither the vocational nurse nor the professional nurse can leave their patients. Both tend to shun being publicly outspoken or militant. Thus, they join professional associations and seek improvements in their employment conditions quietly. They do not join trade unions or contemplate industrial action.

The idea of vocation may also be necessary in order to continue doing some of the very unsavoury tasks that nurses are called on to perform. In other words, it can act as a protection against the realities of nursing work. It is noteworthy that many of the learners, both students and pupils, talked about the need for a vocation while older and more experienced nurses less often referred to it. It is, after all, the learners who have to do battle with many of the unsavoury basic tasks of nursing. Nevertheless, in conversations with nurses of all grades the need for or the importance of vocation was mentioned frequently. Little reference to this aspect was made in the questionnaires.

Vocation emphasizes personal characteristics, whereas the professional emphasizes the skill and training needed to nurse effectively. Professionals rely on expertise not the personality of the nurse. The personal characteristics held to be so important by the vocationals tend to be those normally associated with women. Caring, nurturing, kind, loving and supportive, the 'good nurse' looks suspiciously like the 'good woman'. For many nurses, in accepting this view of the good nurse they were implicitly rejecting the view of nurses as skilled, efficient and highly-trained. The two views of the nurse do not always sit happily together. Thus, there is a distrust and condemnation of nurses who 'sit in the office' and who do not leave the paperwork in order to be with the patients. The idea of vocation is often accompanied by a repeated emphasis on the need for discipline and obedience. Both discipline and obedience are firmly inculcated into nurses as they go through their training — both in the school of nursing and on the wards. The combination of obedience and discipline ensures a quiescenct and relatively unquestioning workforce. Such a workforce has learned its place in the health care team and in particular it does not question the status quo. It is a workforce which can easily be manipulated and contained.

At the same time, there was a frequently expressed rejection of the 'academic', reflecting again the dominance of a vocational perspective. Many nurses adopt an anti-academic stance. Nurses are 'born not made' is the clarion call which acts to give graduate nurses and other high-fliers a poor reception. (It is perhaps no coincidence that none of the male nurses I talked to expressed the 'born not made' sentiment. Males, unable to lay claim to all the necessary personal characteristics of the nurse with a vocation, may be forced to pursue the 'professional' line.) Yet, as regards some of the UKCC's proposals in Project 2000, it has been asserted that the professionalizing elite has won the day (Robinson, 1986). A great deal of scorn was aimed at the 'clever nurse'. Yet the great majority of nurses would like increased opportunities for further training and for promotion. Partially, this can be explained by a wish to undertake short, specific courses in which there is presumably little apparent theoretical content. At the same time, some nurses may wish to leave 'bedside nursing' and further training may be the solution. Of course, those nurses who see themselves as having learned *their* nursing on the job, may feel that they are safe from contamination by the theoretical. Nevertheless, there appears to be some tension between the wish for further training and distrust for the 'clever' nurse.

The anti-academicism may also reflect the dominance of the medical profession and the attribution to doctors of great technical skill and expertise. In this view the primary role of nurses is to provide care: cleverness is not necessary to be a good carer. In fulfilling this care role, nurses follow doctors' orders, they do not compete with doctors. Thus, in accepting a lowly, handmaiden position under the direction of the medical profession nurses cannot, with any degree of conviction, press too hard for substantial increases in pay.

In turn, this affects the way in which nurses are seen. Although patients rate highly the attentions and kindnesses of nurses, calling them 'angels', the status accorded to nurses falls short of that accorded to members of the medical profession. Of course, at the same time nurses are seen, because they are women, as simply doing what comes naturally to them. Just as nurses reiterate the need for practical rather than academic skills, so the patients mirror this view and fail to appreciate the extent of the skills and expertise which nurses need. It is quite easy for patients to fail to see the level of responsibility which many nurses bear and the stresses under which they work. By extension, the contribution which good nursing makes to patient care can be undervalued. At the same time, in order to maintain the patients' trust in the doctor, nurses are taught to be silent in the face of rudeness, insults and general lack of respect from some doctors. In their silence, nurses acquiesce to the system in which they are the doormats.

The rejection of the 'clever nurse' has further repercussions. Other semi-professions who have succeeded in their claims for reasonable levels of pay (and more successfully claims for professional status) have accepted the need for a high level of education and technical expertise. Thus, radiographers, physiotherapists and others have not adopted an anti-academic stance. There is no assumption that a good radiographer, for example, needs little academic training. In adopting an anti-academic view, nurses deny the need for a good level of education in nursing. Nurses' constant stress on the practical nature of the job emphasizes the physical rather than the intellectual aspects of nursing. The prevalent belief that nursing cannot be taught but only learned through experience again downgrades the intellectual requirements of nursing. The responsibility and the skills called for from nurses are not recognized.

In putting others first and not complaining, nurses also denigrate one another. They do not sympathize with their colleagues. The needs of colleagues are easily forgotten or played down especially when the patients are so visibly much more in need of care and attention. The most bitter complaint of nurses is of bitchiness, of being unable to trust colleagues — whether senior, junior or of the same rank. Tongues lash, gossip prevails, reputations for being a trouble-maker are established. Because they do not respect themselves, they do not respect those who are like them: their colleagues. In this way nurses can be their own worst enemy. Because anger is not expressed outside their own ranks, it implodes. The fear of being the focus of this anger acts to reinforce the discipline so assiduously taught during training. 'Shut up and put up' is the message. Indeed, it seems as though nurse training has been designed to disable nurses. In being taught to be obedient, well-disciplined, and unquestioning it is perhaps not surprising that nurses find it hard to speak out. Nurses' silence and quiescence act to reinforce the system of control. Their silence has allowed those further up in the nursing hierarchy to continue to adopt an authoritarian stance quite out of keeping with changes in the wider society. The 'unresponsive' management hierarchy is rarely challenged in a coordinated way by its more junior nursing colleagues. The well-known dislike of 'trouble-makers' — those who do speak out and question or complain — ensures that the less acquiescent do not rise. The hierarchy within nursing seeks recruits to its ranks from amongst those nurses who do not rock the boat. In this way a conservative and backward-looking nursing hierarchy can be perpetuated. Of course there are brave souls who try to effect changes and there is room for change. But any change is within severe limits. To incur one's colleagues' wrath ensures that one's plans or innovations are not supported. Thus attempts to effect changes must work within the system and slowly — the system itself is not challenged.

The learned response not to speak out and not to complain is reinforced in everyday contacts with senior nurses. Thus, the authoritarian nature of the nursing hierarchy acts to inhibit nurses in giving loud voice to demands for improvements in promotion prospects or other employment conditions. In accepting the status quo, nurses ensure they continue to occupy a subordinate and undervalued place in the health care team.

Issues of gender rank highly in explaining the position of nurses and the situation within nursing. As noted earlier, the good nurse is remarkably similar in character to the good woman. The hierarchy in nursing is very much female-dominated. Even although men rise through the ranks to the top very much more quickly than women, they are still in the minority. Nursing is, above all, a woman's world. Yet, many of the views adopted by nurses have much in common with misogynistic attitudes found amongst some members of the medical profession. Nurses fail to give sufficient credit to their colleagues. They fail to give support. Instead, the very antithesis of a supportive environment seems to exist. The 'bitchy' atmosphere reported by nurses is a stereotype of the problems of women working together. This atmosphere has nothing to do with women working together. The bitchy atmosphere is in reality a reflection of the unsupportive hierarchical system within which nurses work. Unfortunately a bitchy atmosphere, full of distrust and gossip, is self-perpetuating. It is a closed circle out of which it is difficult to break. Only if the assumptions which underpin so much of nursing practice are challenged, can positive steps be taken to improve it. Thus nurses need to stand back coolly and appraise their contribution to health care, and to accord their work and their colleagues the respect they deserve. Nurses need correspondingly to challenge the misogynistic views which enjoy some popularity amongst nurses.

The need for a supportive environment for nurses cannot be overstated. Nurses are taught to present at all times a smiling, reassuring face to the patients. The calm face that greets each patient in the morning has to cope with a lack of respect from employers, from medical and other colleagues in the health care team, and from other nurses. It is little wonder that nurses report that theirs is a very stressful job, making great emotional demands which spill over into their leisure hours affecting their families and friends. Nurses need all the support they can get.

But the stresses of nursing are exacerbated by recent governments' economic policies regarding the NHS. Underfunding of the health service is not new, and it is not confined to the present government. However, the effects of many years of underfunding are now becoming all too apparent. Nurses feel themselves to be extremely overworked. The overwork is seen as coming primarily from being understaffed. Added to the hampered aspirations for training, promotion, careers, etc., this understaffing has been intolerable. It means that learners are pushed into situations where they have to take on too much responsibility and have little attention given to their needs for training and support. It means that nurses have to live with and accept a lowering of standards in patient care. It means that nurses have to work over their normal hours, with no overtime pay and with little real chance of taking time off in lieu. The recent debacle over the regrading of nurses should really not occasion surprise.

However, in 'soldiering on' under trying conditions, nurses continue to receive the admiration and sympathy of the general public. That support is valuable to nurses. It is a support which is reflected in patients' attitudes to nurses. If and when nurses take action of which the public does not approve, then nurses' experience of their work may be negatively affected. This is part of the double bind in which nurses as 'angels' are enmeshed.

The thanks from the job come from the patients. The patients do not see enough of the nurses. The nurses are rushed and in turn they rush the patients. The patients become only too aware of the pressures on nurses: they do not receive the care they once might have done and for which they would be so grateful. Not surprisingly, the positive feedback, the thanks, from patients are less welcome to nurses who know they are prevented from giving of their best. The satisfactions which nurses obtain from their jobs, from helping patients, from being given appreciation of a job well done, are being taken away from them. It is little wonder they leave.

Nursing *is* different to other jobs. Nurses explicitly and implicitly hold to a notion of vocation. The idea of a vocation is an important self-protection for nurses against the demands of the job: the demands on stamina, emotion and stomach. The ideology which helps sustain nursing acts to foster the view that pay, for example, is secondary. In accepting the idea of vocation and service to others, nurses are less able to speak out on their own behalf. It seems that nurses cannot claim to be in nursing for the patients and also state that the money is important. The two seem to be mutually exclusive.

At the same time, nurses do not greatly favour trade unions or industrial action. Nurses learn early in their training not to speak out. An authoritarian approach favoured by many within nursing's hierarchy together with their well known dislike of 'trouble-makers' ensures that nurses know and stay in their place. An acceptance of a subsidiary position within the health care team together with a distrust of the clever nurse, do not add weight to demands for greater status or levels of pay.

While our research has managed to address some of the ways in which the idea of 'vocation' affects nursing it has not sought to discover if the belief is waning in influence. From the picture presented by the mass media over fairly recent pay demands and discontent over the re-grading of nurses, it does appear that nurses are becoming more vocal. Whether this picture is merely a fiction of the mass media would need careful and detailed investigation. Our interviews were completed by the summer of 1987 — the situation is likely to continue changing.

There are implications for the future of nursing in the tension between the vocational and professional views. The recommendations of Project 2000 for nurses to be taught in colleges and polytechnics have been approved. The next few years will see these new nurses entering the old system. Substantial resentment of the academically clever nurse may mean that these nurses receive rough treatment when they finally leave the world of education. Thus, the division between the professional and the vocational nurses that has been obscured in recent years is likely to become greater. It may mean that nursing becomes further divided between the technically expert, highly trained nurse and the caring, bedside nurse. If the influence of vocation weakens while a more scientific ethos is adopted, technically and academically competent nurses may enjoy a better relationship with, and be accorded greater status by, members of the medical profession. Yet, it is not clear that rank and file nurses want to pursue the path to professionalization. How can nursing aspire to become a profession when so many of its members shun the credentials which others seek to establish for nursing? If the professional view wins the day in nursing, what will be the reaction from patients? Will patients want their 'angels' back? And, what sort of job satisfaction is the nurse of the future to seek? In short, what will the nurse of the future be like?

References

FRANCIS, B. (1988) 'NHS Nursing: vocation, career or just a job?', University of Lancaster, unpublished paper.

MACKAY, L. (1988) 'The nurses nearest the door', *The Guardian*, 18 January, p. 18.

MACKAY, L. (1988) 'Career Women', *Nursing Times*, 9 March, **84**, 10, pp. 42–4.

MACKAY, L. (1988) 'No Time to Care', *Nursing Times*, 16 March, **84**, 11, pp. 33–4.

MACKAY, L. (1989) *Nursing a Problem*, Milton Keynes, Open University Press.

REDFERN, S. J. (1978) 'Absence and Wastage in Trained Nurses: a selective review of the literature', *Journal of Advanced Nursing*, **3**, pp. 231–49.

ROBINSON, J. (1986) 'Through the minefield — and into the sun?', *Senior Nurse*, **4**, 6, pp. 7–9.

WITZ, A. (1987) *The Spider Legislating for the Fly: Patriarchy and Occupational Closure in the Medical Division of Labour 1858-1940*, University of Lancaster, Ph.D. Thesis.

Acknowledgements

This chapter is based on a study: 'Nurse Recruitment and Wastage', conducted under the general direction of Dr Keith Soothill and supported by the Leverhulme Trust.

4
Nursing and the New Technology

Des McNulty and Fraser McLellan

Introduction

In the latter part of the 1980s, the Government has repeatedly blamed deficiencies in public sector performance on the absence of market pressures which, it argues, allows the public sector to operate in a way which is wasteful and unresponsive to consumer demand (Department of Health, 1989). In order to restore choice and improve efficiency, nationalized industries and public utilities have been or are to be privatized and competition is being introduced into the provision of services such as health and education where, for political reasons, a thoroughgoing privatization is not possible. The introduction of developed budgeting systems, 'internal' markets, compulsory competitive tendering, opting out and other such measures are intended to create conditions under which market pressures can be introduced analogous to those which, in the Government's view, regulate the allocation and utilization of resources in the private sector.

In the health service, the measures proposed in the White Paper 'Working For Patients', together with management restructuring following the Griffiths report, are likely to lead to a significant shift in the balance of control over resources between managers and health professionals. Although in setting out the objectives of management restructuring, management budgeting and the introduction of 'market mechanisms' into the health service emphasis is placed on the need to improve efficiency though the extension of financial control over the use of material rather than human resources, it is widely recognized in the health service that the success of these measures in the Government's terms depends on loosening the stranglehold of the professions. Historically, professionalized occupational groups have exercised a considerable measure of control over the running of the health service (Klein, 1983). Consultants have had a particularly powerful influence over the running of departments and in the allocation of resources.

The nursing profession has maintained controls over key matters such as qualifications for entry, training and standards of practice, together with its own distinct occupational hierarchy, established in the aftermath of the Salmon report in the 1960s. The occupational control which it enjoys falls short of full professional control due to nursing's subordination to medicine, the relative weakness of some of its professional structures and the fact that professional accountability is institutionalized within the organizational structure of the health service (Etzioni, 1969). These characteristics, together with the patriarchal domination to which a predominantly female profession is subject (Gamarnikow, 1978), have led to nursing being described as a semi-profession. Despite the lack of power which is implied by the categorization the fact that nursing is organized and recognized as a profession within the health care division of labour remains significant. In the context of the consensual, corporate decision-making system which is now under threat, nursing has been able to retain a considerable degree of control over the management of the nursing function in the health service.

Until recently, professionalization within the health service has limited the scope for rationalization of work practices. The professional can always appeal to specialist knowledge and responsibility when professional control and autonomy are threatened, preventing managers without professional qualifications from enforcing decisions in matters which are defined as within the exclusive competence of the professional. Sensitive though both managers and politicians are to the dangers of being held responsible for decisions which affect the treatment and care of patients, the introduction of new criteria of efficiency will intensify pressure on hospital managers to exercise tighter control over resource allocation and encourage them systematically to utilize comparative data as a means of establishing budgetary discipline over departmental managers, consultants and other health professionals in management or supervisory positions, without overtly interfering in professional matters. The occupational control exercised by the weaker professions or semi-professions such as nursing is especially vulnerable to this drive for efficiency.

Organizational and technical change are closely intertwined in the reorganization of the health service associated with the new style of management. Changes in the management of the health service are dependent on the use of information technology to monitor resource use and performance standards. Recognizing a vast potential market, vendors of computer hardware and software have been designing systems which are intended to meet the requirements of health service managers and there has been a massive growth in the use of information technology within the health service in the last five years. There is a danger that the attitudes of nurses and other groups of professional workers towards the introduction of information technology would be conditioned by the use made of it by management.

However our research in two hospitals where new technology was being introduced showed that there was an awareness on the part of nurse managers and many ordinary nurses of the need to become involved in the design and implementation of technical systems if the nursing profession is to respond effectively to the challenges it faces. Alongside suspicion about the purposes for which new technology is being introduced, and resentment at the availability of resources for computerization when nurses have expressed concern at shortages of resources for patient care, there was a positive and optimistic attitude about the potential usefulness of new technology. At one of the two hospitals the system which was being introduced was designed explicitly for use by nurses. The participation of nurses in the development of this system and the reasons offered for professional involvement illustrate that at least certain groups within the nursing profession are seeking to use information technology to advance their interests and those of the wider profession. The adoption of this positive strategy indicates an awareness of the importance of ensuring that nurses' information requirements are met and their vital interests protected in the design and use of information technology based systems.

Organizational and Technical Change within the Health Service

Sociological research into the effects of the introduction of information technology (IT) on occupations has been concentrated on the private sector; in manufacturing, retailing, distribution and financial services. Here market pressures and profit orientated notions of efficiency have been major factors stimulating and governing the pattern of technical change. The labour process approach, which identifies managerial attempts to secure more effective control over the labour process as the driving force behind technological innovation and associated organizational change (Blackburn *et al.*, 1985), has been criticized by those who reject the idea of a single capitalist rationality and stress the importance of political processes taking place within the organization. The technical and social organization of work is seen as an outcome of choice and negotiation. Managers make 'strategic choices' in determining whether or how new technology is to be introduced which may be based on a variety of considerations among which enhanced control over labour may not be the most important factor (Child, 1985; McLoughlin and Clark, 1988). For example, Batstone (1987) indicates that the reduction of administrative costs rather than the fact that new technology would enable the substitution of labour and restrict worker autonomy was the decisive influence in decisions made by an insurance company to introduce an IT based system, while in an engineering firm the crucial factor was improved product quality. Also, the use of technology is subject to both formal and informal negotiation (Wilkinson, 1983). Managers are not the sole arbiters of the direction and outcome of techno-logical and organizational change, even though they may be the most sig-nificant actors in the process. Account has to be taken of the attitude of all parties, their relative strengths and weaknesses, the clarity with which they identify their objectives and interests and the vigour with which they are willing to pursue them. For management, securing the consent and co-operation of the workforce is a vital determinant of the success or failure of the introduction of new technological systems.

While many of the analyses developed in the context of the private sector can be applied in the public sector, attention has to be paid to the separate conditions under which technical change takes place. The external stimulus for technological and organizational change provided in the private sector by the market, or, as labour process theorists would suggest, by the underlying structural tendencies of capitalism, are substituted for in the public sector by political and financial pressures emanating from Govern-ment. The Government's ability to set the pattern of administrative control of the health service, exercise control over expenditure and lay down its own priorities have had a significant influence on the nature and scope of techno-logical innovation within the health service. However, the effects of this are not uniform. Earlier in the decade, government policy of controlling costs to the Treasury by maintaining tight budgetary constraints acted as a brake on the introduction of new technology. More recently, recognition of the role of new technology in helping to ensure more effective management of resources and hence greater 'value for money' has ensured that funds have been made available for technological innovation and especially for pilot projects associated with the introduction of resource management and management information systems.

In the health service, managerial strategic choices are thus made in the context of government policies which set parameters for the direction and broad pattern of change. This should not be taken to mean that the outcome of technical change is entirely in accordance with government plans or wishes. As in the private sector, technical change is influenced by 'inter-vening processes and actions' (Child, 1985). Within the orbit of the region, health district or individual hospital, different groups are likely to be struggling to influence the decision-making process to secure control or compete for resources. Technical and organizational change within hospitals is contested by various parties with conflicting aims, ambitions and rivalries. To succeed in meeting the requirements laid down by Government, management needs to secure the consent of key occupational groups. Consent may be difficult to achieve. The complexity and scale of the health service, the organization of significant sections of the workforce into professions and public interest in health care provision can make it very difficult for hospital or area management to resolve conflicts arising from technical and organizational change through local formal and informal negotiation processes similar to those which might take place in industry or commerce.

The wider political debate about the future of the health service, and the way in which professional associations have sought to challenge the policies of Government, has had a considerable bearing on the attitudes of nurses and doctors towards technical and organizational change. There is a widespread fear that the ethos of public provision according to need which has underpinned health provision in the UK will be undermined if the Government's economic philosophy is enshrined in new allocative procedures and managerial practices. This has fanned concern over the introduction of new managerial and budgetary systems, influencing attitudes to the introduction of new technology, especially where it appears to be associated with the extension of managerial control. Some health professionals, feeling that their professional judgment is being subordinated to budgetary considerations, may feel disinclined to cooperate fully with the introduction of IT based management information systems. Any refusal on the part of health professionals to cooperate is potentially highly damaging from the point of view of management because systems are data dependent and increasingly nurses and doctors as well as administrative staff are required to feed in information.

It is unlikely that doctors and nurses could or would operate a collective tactic of non-cooperation. In combatting the white paper proposals the strategy of both the British Medical Association representing doctors and the Royal College of Nursing representing the majority of nurses is to try to exert political pressure on Government. Reluctance on the part of the professional associations to take conventional forms of industrial action which could be construed as damaging to patients is both a strength and a weakness. It helps to preserve public support for the profession and brings an added moral dimension to the profession's negotiating position but it entails a reliance of the political acceptability of the professional case, either to Government or to the wider public. Professional bodies are not always successful when using this approach. In 1986 the RCN's campaign against the Griffiths proposals which, it argued (King, 1986), would lead to the removal of a nursing input from managerial decision-making and the possible loss or reduction of professional control over key aspects of patient care, was not notably successful in securing changes in government policy. The medical profession has enjoyed wide public support in its more recent campaign against the White Paper. However, despite the political sophistication and organizational strength of the BMA, which is reputed to have spent in excess of £1 million on its campaign, the Government has indicated that it intends to go ahead with its proposals for hospitals to be allowed to opt out. Ultimately success depends on the responsiveness of policy makers either to the logic of the case being made or the effectiveness of the pressure being brought to bear.

The conflict between the Government and the medical profession may turn out to be a matter of sound and fury, signifying nothing more than a jockeying for concessions on the part of the latter. If the history of the NHS teaches any precedents, they are that consultants are well able to defend their own interests and frequently do so at the expence of other occupational groups. It cannot be assumed that changes in management approach once implemented will be entirely to the advantage of managers or are mainly at the expense of the professions. Although the introduction of resource management may give managers greater power relative to health professionals, the performance of managers will also be measured by means of performance indicators. The principal victims of the drive for efficiency through technical and organizational change are likely to be ancillary workers who because of their lack of formal responsibility for the treatment and care of patients have much less scope for exercising control over the trajectory of organizational and technical change than professionals.

Nurses are in a middle position, protected by their professional status. Lacking the political or organizational muscle openly to resist change, the nursing profession might seek to influence and exercise some measure of control over it through processes of formal and informal negotiation with management which is seeking consent and cooperation from professional groups in order to introduce new technical and organizational systems. It is our contention that the way in which information technology is to be used, and in particular the design of technical systems, will become an increasingly important matter in relation to the protection and promotion of professional interests. For the nursing profession the adoption of such a strategy is not without difficulties. The interests of the profession may not be held entirely in common. Involvement of some professionals in system design and implementation may not secure the interests of the profession as a whole. Nurses who are coopted by management on to project teams to initiate or co-ordinate the development of new technical systems may end up identifying with the problems of management rather than representing the interests of the majority of the profession. However, the strong commitment which most nurses have to professional values makes it unlikely that they will completely redefine themselves as managers rather than members of a profession. The benefit of such an approach is that the involvement of professionals can facilitate the design and implementation of systems which meet the information needs of professionals and are accepted by them as well as meeting requirements of managers.

Case Studies

Over the last two years research has been undertaken at two sites in Scotland where IT based systems are being introduced. At one hospital, identified henceforth as Hospital A, a nursing information system was introduced from November 1985. At the second hospital, Hospital B, a hospital information system was introduced in 1986. Hospital B was designated as a pilot site for the introduction of resource management and this influenced, although it did not dictate, the choice of the information system. The two systems are sharply contrasting even though they fulfil some of the same functions. The information system at Hospital B is a hospital-wide patient administration system. Most patient records are contructed on admission by medical records staff but in some wards these administrative tasks are carried out by nurses. The nursing information system at Hospital A involves nurses in entering information on patients for administrative use but its prime purpose is to establish a nursing care plan which can be continually updated and printed out from the ward terminal. Thus both systems exist to provide patient records but whereas Hospital B's system is a general administrative record capable of being used to aid resource management within the hospital, Hospital A's nursing information system is a dedicated system providing the nurse at the point of care delivery with an easily read, comprehensive and unambiguous statement of patient care.

The system installed at Hospital B is essentially a management system even though there are a variety of modules to suit different hospital functions. As a result, nurses are in a weak position in negotiating how the system should be used and in suggesting modifications in the design of the system so that it meets their particular needs. Of the twenty-seven nursing staff interviewed in wards where the system had been installed, only one, a senior sister, was involved personally in the design of the system. The fact that the computer at ward level was restricted to administrative tasks was a source of frustration for many of the nursing staff who felt that it did not serve their professional requirements. This is not to suggest that it was of no use to nurses. The system allowed some improvements to the quality of records and saved time spent on multiple entry of basic information about patients. It also provided senior nurse managers with better quality information on matters such as bed occupation and patient flows through different wards on which they could base calculations regarding staffing levels. Several nurses, however, pointed to the fact that the capacities of the system were greater than those presently being used and expressed the hope that once the system was fully installed it would serve their professional needs.

There were some differences between wards which reflected differences in the task and position of sections of the nursing staff. The nurses in the maternity unit had a more positive attitude towards the system despite the fact that it was of limited use to their clinical requirements. Other nurses, such as those involved in coronary care, felt that the system was more time-consuming and distracted them from patient care. One reason for this appeared to be that midwives and nurses in the maternity unit defined their task in a different way — they saw record-keeping and information-gathering as an intrinsic and necessary part of their work both in identifying possible clinical problems and ensuring effective administration. For other nurses record-keeping was an added burden which could not be delegated to more junior staff by trained ward staff. Indeed the majority of nursing staff in Hospital B saw the computer system as extraneous to their job which was providing patient care, and were resentful of the resources being put into it. Of those who agreed that computerization was desirable many spoke of the inevitability of its introduction and expressed the hope that in the long run computers would be of benefit to patient care.

The nursing information system at Hospital A is not simply an administrative system although it could readily be used to provide information about the use of resources, both nursing and material. It was intended by those people from a variety of professional backgrounds involved in its original design and development to support what was seen as good nursing practice. In the course of their work some members of the project team produced papers providing insights into the effects the nursing information system was intended to have on nursing practice. It was argued firstly that a nursing information system could improve nurse to nurse communication within and between wards. Nursing staff coming on duty were able to ascertain at once from the computerized care plan those areas which required their attention. The nursing plan was entered as part of the nursing record which could be transferred with the patient as the patient moved from ward to ward or was discharged from the hospital in favour of community base care. It was argued that the nursing information system improved accountability and supervision by simplifying the task of the charge nurse in monitoring care provision and allowing the record to be updated at the point of implementation of the care plan. Nurses would spend less time on clerical work, freeing more time to be spent on patient care and in making assessments of patients' psychological and social needs.

The nursing information system could potentially be developed as a decision support system for the provision of care on a patient rather than a task-orientated basis. The establishment of a standardized nursing record through the system would enable the 'spontaneous' adoption of patient-orientated methods of care and promote an improvement in the quality of nursing care thereby. In practice the preferred strategy in introducing the nursing information system at Hospital A was to adopt an incremental approach, introducing and developing the system gradually over a specified period. This meant that the system in use at the time when our research was being carried out was still essentially a task-orientated nursing order system which was based on a pre-formatted nursing order list. Those implementing the system were attempting to use the development period to train staff to the point where the system could be customized and the 'activities of living' model of nursing practice could be incorporated, a step which has since been taken.

It is interesting that the technological system appeared to lend itself more easily to a task-based approach where the nursing record provided an individualized checklist of tasks for each patient rather than as a framework which nurses could use for planning care. Professional ideology has been shifting away from a task-orientated approach and towards the adoption of the idea of the 'nursing process' to emphasize the need for nurses to exercise professional judgment using nursing skills and knowledge. This might appear to be compromised by the introduction of the undeveloped nursing information system. But although the nursing information system may in one sense have involved a step backwards, the creation of a decision support system designed for, and to a large extent by, nurses would more than compensate in the future.

Reactions to the use of information technology were consistenly more positive amongst nurses using the dedicated system in Hospital A than they were at Hospital B. Probing the reasons for this, we concluded that these could not be accounted for purely in terms of the greater appropriateness of the nursing information system in relation to nursing practice. In reaction to comments made in interviews by nurse managers associated with the introduction of the nursing information system we identified the existence of a sub-group within the profession, whom we came to describe as 'committed experts'. These are people who have both a strong personal vested interest, in terms of advancement, in the development and use of new technology by nurses and who maintain a strong commitment to the profession. The use of the term 'committed experts' refers to the existence of a network within the profession of nurse managers as well as others who have developed expertise in the design, implementation and use of technologically based systems. The growth of user groups, support organizations such as the British Computer Society Nursing Specialist Group, as well as the appearance in nursing journals of articles dealing specifically with information technology applications are evidence of the growing interest in information technology and the emergence of 'specialists' within the profession. It should be stressed, however, that committed experts are not computer specialists; their expertise lies primarily in nursing. They are predominantly in managerial or research positions within the profession and have acquired practical knowledge of system use and, perhaps through contact with fellow users, awareness of the potential uses and applications of information technology in nursing.

The committed experts we interviewed at Hospital A communicated to nurses operating the system their perception of the advantages for nursing in using information technology to advance professional claims and to defend professional control. They shared a collective desire to ensure that technical change did not undermine the professional status of nursing relative to the other professions within the health care division of labour. Acute anxiety was expressed at the possibility of technical change affecting both preferred standards of service delivery and professional control over the definition of appropriate tasks and the proper means for their accomplishment. If nursing was to retain its professional autonomy and to make any advances then it should act either to establish its own technological systems or attempt to build its specific information requirements into systems for general use within hospitals so that current areas of control would not be jeopardized by the introduction of systems which were designed to meet solely the requirements of management or other professional groups. The experiences of staff at Hospital B illustrate both the frustrations of being expected to use a system which has no obvious pay-off for nursing and the consequences of nurses becoming fully involved only in the implementation stage.

Although the introduction of a nursing information system would not entirely prevent management from attempting to dictate working practices, the establishment of a technical system, in which occupational practices which reflect dominant professional philosophies are enshrined and which incorporates professionally established standards and procedures, makes it more difficult for management to justify intervention. A clear advantage of a proactive strategy is that the profession is seen to be playing its part in policy decisions regarding the future development of information systems. To that extent the involvement of nurses in the design of technical systems and the attempt to use technology to improve professional practice improve the capacity of the profession to direct the path of technical change, rather than technology becoming a means of enforcing managerial control.

Conclusion

A key factor in the maintenance of occupational control is the extent to which practitioners are able to determine what tasks or problems their skills are able to resolve and the 'best way' of employing those skills. Unlike most professions, nursing exists in an elaborate, highly technical division of labour among a number of occupations ordered both by specialization and authority. In particular, the nursing profession exists in a subordinate relation to that of medicine, a relationship cemented by patriarchy. Despite this, nurses have secured over the years some considerable degree of control over the performance of tasks and the management of the nursing function. Managerial restructuring, resource management and the introduction of information technology appear to place this occupational control in jeopardy.

One aspect of this is the attempt by management to establish criteria through which the characteristics of various work tasks can be identified separately from the way in which professionals carry them out. Whereas in many occupational fields the product of technical work is normally separate from the work processes involved in its production, allowing its quality and characteristics to be judged independently from the individual competence of producers, in health care it has in the past been difficult to separate service provision from its consumption (see Larson, 1977); the 'product' of nursing was healthy people. Jamous and Peloille (1970) argue that the crucial factor in occupational control is the ratio between 'indetermination' and 'technicality'. Roughly defined, indetermination refers to those aspects of a particular task which cannot be codified and rendered subject to rules and procedures. It comprises those areas of work which rely on the individual skills and capacities of workers, consequently distancing the accomplishment of certain tasks from the scrutiny of managers, patients and even other professionals. Technicality, on the other hand, refers to procedures that can be passed on in the form of rules. Where the ratio of indetermination to technicality is high, practitioner control is strong; conversely if the ratio is low practitioner control is weak.

Despite its subordinate position with respect to medicine, nursing fits to a considerable extent into the former category. Nurses need to maintain a range of skills in order to deal with contingencies that might arise — indeed, aspects of nursing could be described as 'crisis management'. Although much of nurses' work is predictable and routine, much is not; and hence is not easy to measure or to programme. The discretionary powers which nurses possess in the field of patient care, although less than and subordinate to medicine, are significant as a barrier to any prospective 'Taylorization'. One of the few ways in which the nursing profession can protect itself against the encroachment of managerial control is to become involved in the design of technical systems to ensure that professional standards are being maintained and that the systems correspond to professional needs. Yet in doing so, there is a tendency for nursing to become rule governed and to reduce the indeterminacy/technicality ratio. The net effect could be the segmentation of the profession so that qualified, technically competent staff carry out all non-routine work while less qualified staff perform routine tasks, having received their instructions and being supervised via a technological interface. This possibility is not unique to nursing, but the organizational upheaval in the health service and acute staffing and recruitment shortages anticipated in the 1990s may trigger change. To put this final point into perspective, in 1983 the NHS recruited 43 per cent of the available suitably qualified women entrants into the labour market; by 1993 the proportion required will be 62 per cent (BMJ, 1989). If implemented, Project 2000, which aims to alter the balance between education and in-service training, will exacerbate rather than alleviate shortages in the 1990s. It may be that demographic factors will provide the greatest stimulus to further technical and organizational change.

References

BARLEY, S. R. (1986) 'Technology as an occasion for structuring: evidence from observations of CT scanners and the social order of radiology departments', *Administrative Science Quarterly*, **31**, pp. 78–108.

BATSTONE, E. (1987) *New Technology and the Process of Labour Regulation*, Oxford, Clarendon Press.

BELLABY, P. and ORIBABOR, P. (1980) 'Determinants of Occupational Strategies Adopted by British Hospital Nurses', *International Journal of Health Services*, **10**, 2, pp. 291–309.

BLACKBURN, P. *et al.* (1985) *Technology, Economic Growth and the Labour Process*, London, Macmillan.

BRITISH MEDICAL JOURNAL (1989) 'Running Out of Staff for the NHS', *British Medical Journal*, **299**, 1 July.

CARPENTER, M. (1978) 'Managerialism and the Division of Labour in Nursing', in DINGWALL, R. and MCINTOSH, J. (Eds) *Readings in the Sociology of Nursing*, Edinburgh, Churchill Livingstone.

CHILD, J. (1985) 'Managerial Strategies, New Technology and the Labour Process', in KNIGHTS, D. *et al.* (Eds) *Job Redesign: Critical Perspectives on the Labour Process*, Aldershot, Gower.

CHILD, J. *et al.* (1984) 'Microelectronics and the quality of employment in services', in MARSTRAND, P. (Ed.) *New Technology and the Future of Work and Skill*, London, Frances Pinter.

CLARK, J. *et al.* (1988) *The Process of Technical Change: New Technology and Social Choice in the Workplace*, Cambridge, Cambridge University Press.

DEPARTMENT OF HEALTH (1989) *Working For Patients*, London, HMSO.

DEPARTMENT OF HEALTH AND SOCIAL SECURITY STEERING GROUP ON HEALTH SERVICES INFORMATION (Chair Mrs E. Korner) (1984) *A Report on the Collection and Use of Financial Information in the National Health Service*, London, HMSO.

DINGWALL, R. and LEWIS, P. (1983) *The Sociology of the Professions*, London, Macmillan.

ETZIONI, A. (1969) *Semi-Professions and their Organisation*, New York, Free Press.

FARDELL, J. (1989) 'Fighting Together', *Nursing Times*, **85**, 11, 15 March.

FRANCIS, A. (1986) *New Technology at Work*, Oxford, Oxford University Press.

FREIDSON, E. (1970) *Profession of Medicine*, New York, Harper and Row.

GAMARNIKOW, E. (1978) 'Sexual Division of Labour — The Case of Nursing', in KUHN, A. and WOLPE, A. M. (Eds) *Feminism and Materialism*, London, Routledge and Kegan Paul.

JAMOUS, H. and PELOILLE, B. (1970) 'Changes in the French University-Hospital System', in JACKSON, J. A. (Ed.) *Professions and Professionalisation*, Cambridge, CUP.

JOHNSON, T. (1972) *Professions and Power*, London, Macmillan.

KING, M. M. (1986) 'Revolt of Angels', *The Guardian*, 29 January.

KLEIN, R. (1983) *The Politics of the National Health Service*, London, Longman.

KNIGHTS, D. and WILLMOTT, H. (1986) *Gender and the Labour Process*, Aldershot, Gower.

LARSON, M. S. (1977) *The Rise of Professionalism*, California, University of California Press.

MCLOUGHLIN, I. and CLARK, J. (1988) *Technological Change at Work*, Milton Keynes, Open University Press.

MASON, A. and MORRISON, V. (Eds) (1985) *Walk Don't Run*, London, King's Fund Publishers.

SCHOLES, M. *et al.* (1983) *The Impact of Computers on Nursing*, Amsterdam, Elsevier.

STRAUSS, A. *et al.* (1973) 'The Hospital and its Negotiated Order, in SALAMAN, G. and THOMPSON, K. (Eds) *People and Organisations*, London, Longman.

WEBSTER, F. and ROBINS, K. (1986) *Information Technology: A Luddite Analysis*, Norwood, NJ, Ablex Publishing Corporation.

WILKINSON, B. (1983) *The Shopfloor Politics of New Technology*, London, Heinemann.

5
Professional Status and Managerial Tasks: Feminine Service Ideology in British Nursing and Social Work

Maria Lorentzon

Altruistic service has traditionally been associated with the role of women. Its roots have been viewed as partly biological and linked to motherhood. 'Nature' has been seen to ordain this pattern of female function, which provides the nurturing and often hidden elements cementing the nuclear family and by extension society at large. This 'ideal type' of femininity, radically challenged by feminists, formed part of the inspiration of female Victorian reformers of health and welfare institutions, who may be viewed as the pioneers of modern nursing and social work.

The main focus in this chapter is on consideration of nursing and social work as numerically female-dominated occupations, imbued with a service ideology which might be described as essentially 'feminine' in its original inspiration, but which is increasingly challenged by masculine rationality within bureaucratic health and welfare institutions. Femininity and masculinity are viewed as Weberian 'ideal types' in this context and issues of managerialism and professionalism are raised in the analysis of relevant documents to highlight important aspects of the central debate on gender roles within what Etzioni (1969) describes as 'semi-professions'. Arising from this 'theoretical take-off point' consideration of theories on professionalization is implied. The traditional 'trait theories' on pro-fessionalization as described by Johnson (1972) form the foundation for the debate. The research centres primarily on the examination of official documents published between 1959 and 1983 which are concerned with nursing and social work in Britain, but reference is also made to Victorian sources as noted above. The documents concerned with nursing are the Platt Report (1964), dealing with nurse education and propagating separation of this sector from the NHS service establishment, the Salmon Report (1966) which claims to provide a rational career structure for senior nursing staff, the Briggs Report (1972) which consolidates the Salmon philosophy and sets out to examine the roles and educational requirements of nurses and midwives and the Nurses, Midwives and Health Visitors Act (1979) which confirms the Briggs findings and, lastly, the Griffiths Report (1983) which deals with the broader aspects of NHS management, affecting nurses profoundly as will be demonstrated in this discussion. The reports relating to social work are the Younghusband Report (1959) which explores the role, recruitment and training of social workers, the Seebohm Report (1968) which investigates the wider field of social services, the Barclay Report (1982) which sets out to review the role and tasks of social workers and, finally, the Parsloe Report (CCETSW Documents 20:1 and 20:2) (1983) which proposes radical change in the pattern of social work education. Professional journals, which are thought to reflect rank and file opinion in nursing and social work, are explored in order to chart the response to the reports listed above. Among others, they include the *Nursing Times, Nursing Mirror, Social Work Today* and *Community Care*.

The main thrust of the discussion is oriented towards the period between 1959 and 1983, but in order to ground the debate within the historical tradition of nursing and social work, it will be necessary to 'step back' briefly into the nineteenth century. In examining historical references to nursing and social work pioneers, it is important to separate image and reality as far as possible. Recent historians of nursing, including Smith (1982) and Prince (1984), have gone a long way towards demythologizing Nightingale, 'The Lady of the Lamp', to find beneath the sugared surface 'The Hypochondriac' and 'The Machiavellian Manipulator', as well as the rational social researcher. Likewise, the prevailing 'official' image of the nurse as a self-sacrificing 'angel of mercy' contains within itself both the seeds of the domineering woman, as discussed by Campbell (1984) and the rational careerist following the path staked out in the Salmon Report. Within the sphere of early social work, Octavia Hill dealt with her tenants in the manner of a strict, Victorian mother and contained within herself the same tension between 'hard' and 'soft' personal characteristics as discussed by Roszak and Roszak (1969) in related to gender traits. Likewise, Twining (1898) held what might be described as 'strict views' on social welfare. Authoritarian symbolism has, however, been less marked in social work than in nursing as it is largely without uniforms and other institutional signs, which form part of the traditional, female nursing model.

Consideration of nursing and social work as semi-professions with strong numerical female dominance raises issues which relate to altruism and what might be described as 'feminine professionalism'. The contrast between this form of service ideology as discussed by Halmos (in Heraud, B. (1981)) and Lorentzon (1987) and structural professionalization, based on autonomy and institutional power and described by Johnson (1972) and Freidson (1970) distinguishes semi or feminine professionalism from the traditional professionalism of male dominated disciplines, such as medicine and law. While the professional core activities of medical and legal practice can be exercised even at a senior level, nurses, social workers and other semi-professionals tend to become increasingly involved in management as they climb the career ladder. This was noted by Etzioni and the selected reports on nursing and social work support this theory.

In analyzing documentary material it is assumed that the notion of professional structure according to the 'trait theory' (Johnson, 1972) is a viable concept, although by no means the only approach to professionalization. The model of managerialism is that of Weber's 'ideal type' of rational bureaucracy.

The Younghusband Report (1959) supports the right of social workers to remain in professional practice without being penalized in terms of salary and status. Barclay (1982) also recommends that social workers should break with traditional management thinking associated with giving higher status to managerial than to social work practice roles. Similarly, a need to defend the professional aspects of social work practice was identified following the Seebohm-inspired reorganization of social services departments, by ensuring that while social work was to become essentially 'generic', there should also be scope for professional specialization (*Community Care*, 14 September 1977, p. 22). Stronger NHS management was proposed in the Griffiths Report (1983); the consensus model would give way to general management, which was viewed as more efficient. The general reaction to the report by nurses was one of apprehension and it was seen as essential for a substantial number of nurses to become general managers, as their exclusion from these posts would result in 'much of the progress made since Salmon [being] wiped out' (*Nursing Times*, 20 June 1984, p. 3). Fear of being barred from general management posts rather than a reluctance by nurses to undertake these tasks typified their reaction to the Griffiths proposals.

Many reports and journal contributions pointed to a general proliferation of managerial traits and social work. The many-headed monster of post-Seebohm, large scale bureaucracy in social work, was seen to have triplicated the practical chores of practitioners (*Social Work Today*, 6 September 1973, p. 388). Disillusionment with the 'promised land' envisaged through the Seebohm reforms had, six months after their implementation, caused many social workers to long for a return 'to Egypt' (*Social Work Today*, 21 October 1971, p. 31). The Briggs Report was also criticized, in that its proposals for nursing were seen to create an impersonal and over-complicated structure of administration (*Nursing Times*, 8 March 1973, p. 168).

The historical development of nursing within large hierarchical institutions has led to evolution or archaic modes of leadership (Briggs, 1972) and it was hoped that the Salmon structures would achieve the required modernization. The tension between professional and managerial traits and what Parry and Parry (in Heraud, 1981, p. 135) aptly term 'bureau-professionalism', applies in nursing and social work and is discussed with reference to the latter occupation following publication of the Younghusband Report (1959). A writer in *The Almoner* stressed the need for 'economising in the use of trained personnel' (Supplement, January 1960, p. 2). In the wake of the Briggs Report a contributor to the *Nursing Times* spoke of 'the gulf between practitioners and administrators [being] wider than ever' (1972, p. 1073).

The confused ideology of social work was described in *Social Work Today* with reference to the Barclay Committee (1982) which failed to establish 'the values, methods, skill and knowledge' associated with professional social work (13 July, 1982, p. 9). This ambivalence between management and professional practice is resolved by uneasy compromise in the suggestion that both practitioners and managers are engaged in social work (Barclay, 1982). A writer in the *Nursing Mirror* suggested that nurses with a managerial bent would be better off entering hospital management (18 December, 1970, p. 37). The Griffiths Report was seen to have left nurses out in the cold both professionally and in terms of management input (*Nursing Times*, 23 November 1983, p. 10; 2 November 1983, p. 7; *Nursing Mirror*, 2 November 1983, p. 5). Members of professional organizations and statutory bodies were concerned about lack of consultation with nurses (*Nursing Times*, 7 December 1983, p. 19) and one writer described the confused state of nursing in the following terms: 'Like social workers and teachers, nurses belong to what Etzioni calls semi-professions. Essentially this means that professional accountability is to a large extent institutionalised within an organisational structure, a situation not normally found in professions' (*Nursing Times*, 8 August 1984, p. 19).

The interaction between professional and managerial authority in nursing underlies the anxiety about diminution of managerial power within the occupational group. However, Norman Fowler, Secretary of State at the time, reassured nurses that chief nursing officers in district health authorities would continue to have a vital role (*Nursing Times*, 13 June 1984, p. 6); and one nurse, writing in the *Nursing Times*, went further by voicing the view that these senior nurse managers would be ideal candidates for general management (11 July 1984, p. 63). A fitting summary of the semi-professional's position is made by Catherine Hawkins, the only nurse general manager in post in January 1985, who urged nurses to 'sell themselves as managers first and as nurses second' if they wanted to succeed in the post-Griffiths health service (*Nursing Mirror*, 8 August 1984, p. 5).

Rationality within the national health service and social services department hierarchies of the type described by Weber runs like a leitmotif through the recent phases of development. This facet of public service management coexists with, and is frequently seen to stand in opposition to, the factional interests of various occupational groups involved in the multi-disciplinary institutions. The varying power positions of these groups can be referred to in terms of degree of professionalization and it may be assumed that those with 'weaker' professional status will be more likely to succumb to managerial influences as discussed by Etzioni (1969). Both nursing and social work fall into this category. The Salmon and Seebohm Reports both deal with rational management in nursing and social work / social services respectively. The Salmon Committee (1966) pointed to the inefficiency of 'matrons . . . assuming control of services extraneous to nursing' (Salmon, 1966, p. 23) and saw this as detrimental to the overall health service delivery (*Nursing Times*, 11 January 1973, p. 7). The Briggs Committee (1972) later provided the view that Salmon should be 'brought down into the ward' in order to provide rational management at the point of clinical care delivery (*Nursing Times*, 11 January 1973, p. 7). Rationality in social work/social services delivery was also emphasized by the Seebohm Committee (1968), re-iterating the 'demand for a united service' (*Social Work*, October 1968, p. 3). The Parsloe Committee (1983) likewise cast doubt on the virtue of separating social work from social services as a whole (Doc. 20:1, CCETSW (1983), p. 3). However, a management reorganization of that nature might lead to 'a colossal dilution' of trained staff with experienced social workers becoming administrators (*Community Care*, 14 September 1977, p. 22).

The tension between managerial and professional interests is evident above and must be resolved within a rational management model. The Griffiths Enquiry (1983) provided a plan to rationalize the National Health Service in an economic climate of shrinking resources. Opposition from professional and semi-professional groups was strong, especially from nursing, whose members experienced considerable threat from its proposals, both professionally and in terms of management involvement. There was a self-confessed realization of deficiency by nurse managers (*Nursing Times*, 21 December, 1983, p. 4) and the Regional General Manager, Catherine Hawkins, dared to suggest against the majority nurse opinion, that 'the profession had over-reacted to the Griffiths Report' (*Nursing Times*, 15 August 1984, p. 19). She pointed out that industrial managers often take charge over professional workers and also stressed that nurse managers must sell themselves as such. This accords with the theories of Dingwall and Lewis (1983) regarding professionals within bureaucratic institutions.

While evidence of uncomfortable tension between professional and managerial traits is evident in the documentary material, management definitions of function would seem to prevail in senior positions and are strongly defended by nurses in regard to the Griffiths proposals. While a similar tendency prevails in social work, it would seem to be less marked.

Apart from the tendency towards dominance by management definitions over professional theories within semi-professions, it would seem that a particular form of gender division of labour is prone to develop. Thus it would appear that in nursing and social work a disproportional number of men hold managerial/instrumentally oriented posts, whereas women predominate within professional/expressively slanted areas of work. It might be suggested that *'feminine'* rather than *semi*-professionals would be the best description for these workers.

Theories related to separate gender spheres (Ruskin, 1898), male instrumentality versus female expressiveness (Parsons, 1964) and male aggresiveness versus female submissiveness (Goldberg, 1979) are of interest in this context as well as the opposing feminist arguments. The perceived 'femaleness' of nursing and social work is historically enshrined in titles such as 'sister', 'matron' and 'lady almoner' and numerical female dominance in the two occupations has only diminished very gradually from the nineteenth century until the present time. It might be suggested that prevailing nursing and social work ideology is not necessarily 'weak' or semi-professional, although some light is thrown on the question by exploring the difference between established professions, for example medicine and law, and other occupations such as nursing and social work. It could be argued that feminine professionalism operates differently from traditional professionalism and is not simply a diluted version.

The Younghusband Report (1959) refers to a predominance of women in more nurturant and men in more bureaucratic, managerial forms of social work. Welfare officers, who were predominantly male, tended to work in largely administrative settings and these agencies were mainly staffed by workers without formal professional qualifications (Younghusband, 1978, Parts I and II). However, entry to medical social work, which had a higher proportion of female workers, normally necessitated professional training (*op. cit.*, Part I). Reference to 'lady almoners' would seem to denote that most social workers in hospitals and health departments were orginally female (Younghusband, 1959, p. 94). While almoners were normally professionally qualified and employed in 'nurturant', person-centred casework, their original function *was* that of 'financial gate-keeper', ensuring that the 'undeserving' were kept out of voluntary hospitals (Huntington, 1981) and their main task was thus of an administrative/managerial nature. A case-work approach developed gradually, however, with increasing numbers of almoners possessing a professional qualification, as referred to above.

Following the Parsonian model of gender-typing, 'rational/masculine' management methods were encouraged in the Salmon Report by propagating a line management approach (Salmon, 1966, p. 9). In contrast 'fussy/expressive/feminine' forms of authority were criticized in the nursing press, pointing to the matron retaining: 'detailed control of work she purports to delegate and deliberately retaining work which she could well hand over to assistants' (*op. cit.*, p. 24). Matrons must not be allowed to be drawn into management of non-nursing functions (*op. cit.*, p. 23). A male contribution to the *Nursing Mirror* interpreted Salmon as saying that the 'bureaucratic matron' of the past would have to learn the art of delegating power (16 June, 1972, p. 17). He went on to condemn excessive 'femininity' in nurse management, observing that: 'if nurses are to lose the image of fussy, pernickety or unapproachable women without management skills, then they must strive towards the perfection within the terms of reference as set out by Salmon' (*ibid.*).

Views on the subject were mixed, however, and one traditionalist expressed regret that the 'honourable name of matron' would disappear (*Nursing Mirror*, 30 July 1977, p. 9). This discussion about management styles echoes the distinction between paternalist (or in this instance, maternalist/expressive) and autonomous (masculine/rational) forms of authority. The severity of the Victorian, paternalist father could paradoxically be seen mirrored in 'old-fashioned attitudes of some matrons, who rule with a rod of iron' (Briggs, 1972, p. 54). Adoption of the Salmon structure would make 'the present, rigid, authoritarian system merely a hideous memory' (*op. cit.*, p. 162).

Whereas criticism of female leadership in nursing was rife at the time of the Salmon Enquiry, this did not seem to apply to women in leading social work positions. This might be due either to institutional differences between nursing and social work or to the greater 'femininity' of nursing compared to social work applying the criteria of the Parsonian 'ideal type'.

Feminine professionalism is conceived primarily in terms of 'nurturant power', which is relevant to the models of female leadership discussed above. Thus it differs from semi-professionalism in being viewed as *different from* but not necessarily *weaker than* established professionalism. It must be conceded, however, that the 'strength' of the 'feminine professional' does not carry the same legitimacy as that of the 'traditional professional' in Western and indeed almost any known society. The 'power of nurturance' is associated with the 'private' and, in the gender-division of Ruskin, female sphere, whereas the more prestigious public sector is dominated by men and typified in established professions, i.e. medicine and law. This dominance of male values in the West is discussed by many feminist writers, one of whom is Spender (1982). Widespread acceptance of this ideology by both social scientists and the public at large has led to insufficient consideration of 'feminine power' except as 'subservient manipulation' as in the case of Nightingale 'ruling' men from her sick bed (Woodham-Smith, 1951). This may explain the neglect of 'nurturance as power' in general discussions about caring.

The Younghusband Report (1959) points to the roots of contemporary social work in nineteenth-century charitable institutions. Many of these were inspired by female reformers as shown in the writings by Boyd (1982) and Prochaska (1980) about nineteenth-century charitable work and by Twining (1898) recounting her own experiences. The female input to nineteenth-century nursing reform does not need to be recounted at this stage. Nursing was, and perhaps still is to a great extent, essentially 'feminine' in a traditional sense. The notion of 'vocation/dedication' is part of the mother-role on which 'feminine professionalism' is based and is perpetuated in nursing through stress on altruism. This feature, which is often listed as a trait of professionalism, is more marked in 'semi' or 'feminine' professions than in the more traditional equivalents. The Platt Report (1964, p. 10) points to the importance of dedication, and the nurturant side of nursing was a topic of interest for the Briggs Committee (1972), which noted the strong support for direct patient care among nurses in general.

Discussion about the 'dependence' of social work clients in the Barclay Report (1982) centres on the issue of 'paternalism' (*Community Care*, 20 May, 1982, p. 3). It is noteworthy that no mention is made of a female input to dependency relationships of the type described above. Maternalism rather than paternalism would seem an apt description for an ideology established in the main by female reformers in nursing and social work propagating what might be described as 'strict' views on welfare as exemplified in the writings and work of, for example, Octavia Hill and Louisa Twining (Poor Law Conference Reports — W. Midlands (1884) p. 19; South Wales (1901) p. 161; Foreword (1903–1904) pp. viv–xxi). It is interesting to note that an established, male-dominated profession, i.e. medicine, and a female-dominated 'semi-profession' — nursing — have both been likened to social work in terms of exercising social control over clients and patients.

The 'caring/feminine' aspect of social work was not necessarily defined as 'social work proper' by the Barclay Committee (1982). Thus the 'feminine' parts of the practice are degraded without an awareness of the nurturant power inherent in 'tending relationships'. Nurses take on these aspects of *medical* care acting as the 'nurturant' branch of 'scientific' medicine, and are likewise losing 'professional', although not 'feminine professional' status thereby. It would seem from this albeit somewhat speculative discussion that 'professionals' and 'feminine professionals' tend to pursue goals which are sometimes diametrically opposed; that is, the striving for financial recognition and structurally defined professional status stands in opposition to self-sacrificing altruism.

Seebohm (1968) stressed the need to consider authority in social work practice. An important area for discussion in this context is the 'treatment' versus 'punishment' approach in social control. Feminist writers have, generally, assumed that harshness is a masculine trait and Stone (in Fisher (1980) pp. 391–2) saw the increase in flogging as a means of disciplining children and criminals as associated with male ascendancy. The permissive/treatment oriented approach, which became more prevalent in the West in the post Second World War period and blossomed in the 1960s, was associated with defining the criminal/erring child as 'sick and in need of treatment' rather than 'wicked/naughty and deserving of punishment' as discussed by Morris (1974). This model would, using Stone's gender typing, be associated with female, nurturant authority in contrast to male punitiveness. It is, however, debatable whether the latter approach is less harsh in its long-term effects. A criminally insane offender will be given an indeterminate period of treatment in a psychiatric hospital, which may constitute a 'life sentence' unless he is declared 'sane/cured' by the professionals, whereas a 'sane' criminal will normally be 'punished' by enduring a time-limited prison sentence. The situation in countries which retain capital punishment is, of course, different.

Indeterminate sentencing, which took on aspects of the 'treatment mentality' and flourished in the 1960s, is currently opposed by certain sectors in the USA, where a return to punishment is preferred (Clark, D. and Davies, M. in *New Society*, 10 May, 1984, pp. 222–4) and where there are isolated moves to reintroduce corporal punishment as more 'just' and 'humane' than prolonged and indeterminate incarceration (Newman, 1983). In child-rearing there was a similar tendency to label children who misbehaved as 'sick/maladjusted' rather than 'naughty'. This medicalization of 'hyper-active children' in the 1960s bears witness to this tendency. Whereas in the past children who misbehaved received punishment, the permissive treatment approach was to label them as 'medical cases' (Box, 1977).

Whether a case could be made for designating 'therapeutic power' as feminine and 'punitive power' as masculine is a matter for discussion. However, this would seem justified within the context of the present definition of 'feminine professionalism' and arising out of the ideal type of male punitiveness as proposed by Stone above. A more speculative move to suggest that the 'treatment approach' is more powerful than that of 'punishment' and that the former characterizes 'feminine nurturant power' in both nursing and social work, would seem justified. The present data do not, however, give clear support for such a proposition and further research in this area is needed.

Returning again to the examination of reports and professional journals, the perceived femininity of social work pre-1959 was discussed in the Younghusband Report (1959) and the need to recruit more men into the occupation was stressed, especially in the specialist areas where women had hitherto been in the majority (Younghusband, 1959, p. 16). Likewise the Platt Report (1964) rejected exclusive input of 'female expressiveness' in nursing and the notion that qualities of 'the head' were less important to the nurse than those of 'the heart' (*Nursing Times*, 3 July 1964, p. 858). The Salmon Committee (1966) favoured a more substantial input by male nurses whose attitudes were assumed to be more 'managerial' than those of women. Men were seen to be more instrumental in their career orientation (*Nursing Times*, 17 January 1974, p. 68). A case could be made for seeing this as a sign of the greater altruism of women who choose a post for its own sake, whereas men apply more instrumental motives to their career planning.

Following the Salmon Report (1966) doubt was expressed about female nurses coming forward to fill managerial posts (*Nursing Times*, 13 May 1966, p. 625). In the same vein, it was asked whether 'the organisation of woman power for the provision of a bedside nursing service' (*Nursing Times*, 20 May 1966, p. 677) warranted the Salmon system. Evidence of gender typing is apparent in these statements. As if answering the question posed above, the Griffiths Report (1983) seemed to support a return of nurses to the bedside, although this was not explicitly stated. Nurse correspondents feared that they would lose the managerial power gained since the Salmon reorganization, and that, as a consequence, they would be 'pulled back under strong doctor dominance' (*Nursing Mirror*, 23 November, 1983, p. 10). By reverting to a predominantly 'clinical/nurturant' sphere senior nursing personnel would be defined more closely according to the 'feminine/expressive' ideal type in relation to the predominantly male medical profession. Predictably, male nurses reacted strongly against such 'degradation' and Rowden stated defiantly that nursing would not consent to a return to 'managerial and professional subservience' (*Nursing Mirror*, 4 July, 1984, p. 19). It might be argued that nursing is the predominantly caring/female arm of the male-dominated medical profession and that it would thus be in the interest of doctors to reduce the nurse management establishment.

Significantly, the redefinition of social work from being 'women's work' to becoming a 'profession' was applauded in referring to the Seebohm Report (1966) (*Social Work Today*, 16 November, 1976, p. 7). The former might include a notion of 'vocation' and carry traits of 'feminine professionalism', whereas the latter, presumably, approximated social work to the status of medical or legal practice. In the same vein, the most lowly graded social work assistant was described as a 'rounded mum' (*Community Care*, 2 April, 1976, p. 7). The feminine tradition in nursing may account for the fact that male nurses were found to be less well qualified on entering nurse training than their female counterparts, based on findings from a survey quoted by the Briggs Committee (1972) concerning the number of male and female students possessing GCE Advanced Level passes when commencing the course. Whereas 94 per cent of males were without such qualifications, the figure for females was 84 per cent (Briggs, 1972, p. 160). In spite of their generally lower academic standard, a quota system in favour of men entering nursing was proposed (*Nursing Times*, 1 February, 1973, p. 134) as they were seen to offer 'return on training' (Briggs, 1972, p. 121).

The relationship between nursing and social work, on the one hand, and medicine, on the other, has been referred to above and is of interest in the consideration of occupational gender typing. Medical social workers, commenting on the possibility of being separated from medically dominated health care institutions, as proposed in the Seebohm Report (1968), noted that their secondment from area teams would contribute to doctors recognizing 'the proper function of social work' (*Medical Social Work*, September 1968, p. 134). Medical dominance over social work remained the ideal of the older profession, however, and some of the medical evidence to the Barclay Committee reflected this view (*Social Work Today*, 4 May 1982, p. 15). A number of doctors argued in favour of 'medical dominance of social workers as para-professionals' (*Social Work Today*, 13 July, 1982, p. 10). Medical resistance to the rational management model for senior nursing structures, as proposed by Salmon (1966), was typified in the view of a consultant supporting the image of nurses 'with their sleeves rolled up' (*Nursing Times*, 18 February 1971, p. 212). He furthermore rejected the plea by nurses that they should cease doing non-nursing duties. It would seem clear that the preferred role for both nurses and social workers in the view of many doctors was a 'nurturant/maternal' one with the retention of para-medical status.

Many hospital administrators also wished to retain the bedside role for nurses. At the time of the Platt Report (1964) a hospital secretary put aspiring nurse managers firmly in their place, saying: 'we need nurses who nurse and are not too over-educated to attend to a patient' (*Nursing Times*, 3 July 1964, p. 859), and this view was reinforced indirectly in the Griffiths Report (1983) as noted above. Referring to the Salmon structure, the traditional matron's confused notion of 'the true facts of service life' was remarked upon (*Nursing Times*, 22 July 1966, p. 979). Feminine styles of exercising authority were derided as uninformed and irrational.

The Barclay Report dealt with the informal community care sector, conceding that women would be the most likely informal carers (Barclay, 1982, p. 200; *Social Work Today*, 19 October 1982, p. 4). As women predominated in this role, the apparently egalitarian campaign to reduce social work monopoly spelt out the same message to women carers as the Bowlby thesis on 'maternal deprivation' (Bowlby, 1953), that a woman's place is in the home, caring for the young and the helpless. Thus the anti-elitist thrust of the Barclay Report (1982), casting doubt on the qualitative superiority of professional social work over informal caring, was seen to be a double-edged sword, unintentionally reinforcing the 'feminine/nurturant role'.

The original research on which this chapter is based included a substantial section dealing with structures in nursing and social work and the manner in which these have influenced the different development paths in the two occupations. The current emphasis is upon ideological aspects, however, and inclusion of this material would therefore seem inappropriate. It must be noted, however, that social structure and ideology are symbiotically dependent upon each other and a comprehensive analysis of nursing and social work would require discussion of both aspects. Suffice it to say that the research revealed considerable differences between structural arrangements within British nursing and social work in terms of managerial, educational and professional organization and these have had an impact upon the ideology and activities of the two occupations.

Current social and health care policies require increasing cooperation between nursing and social work especially in the areas of child abuse and community care for vulnerable groups, for example, elderly, mentally ill and mentally handicapped people. The areas discussed in this paper demonstrate both similarities and differences between contemporary British nursing and social work. They provide useful background information to aid policy formation in the wake of a report proposing radical reform of nurse education, entitled 'Project 2000' (1986), the rejection of the Parsloe (1983) proposals for social work education, the projected impact of the White Paper 'Working for Patients' (1989) and the second Griffiths Report (1988) on recommended patterns of community care, as we head for the year 2000.

References

BARCLAY, P. (1982) *Social Workers, Their Role and Tasks*, London, National Institute of Social Work.

BOWLBY, J. (1953) *Child Care and the Growth of Love*, Harmondworth, Pelican.

BOX, S. (1977), in National Deviancy Council (Ed.) *Permissiveness and Control*, London, Macmillan.

BOYD, N. (1982) *Josephine Butler, Octavia Hill, Florence Nightingale — Three Victorian Women Who Changed Their World*, London, Macmillan.

BRIGGS, A. (1972) *A Report on the Committee on Nursing*, London, HMSO.

CAMPBELL, A. (1984) *Moderated Love*, London, SPCK.

CLARK, D. and DAVIES, M. (1984) 'The Californian Way of Justice', *New Society*, 10 May, pp. 222–4.

DINGWALL, R. and LEWIS, P. (1983) *The Sociology of the Professions*, London, Macmillan.

ETZIONI, A. (Ed.) (1969) *Semi-professions and Their Organisation*, New York, Free Press.

FREIDSON, E. (1970) *Profession of Medicine*, New York, Free Press.

GOLDBERG, S. (1979) *Male Dominance — The Inevitability of Patriarchy*, London, Abacus.

GRIFFITHS, R. (1983) *Enquiry into NHS Management*, London, DHSS.

GRIFFITHS, R. (1988) *Community Care: Agenda for Action — A Report to the Secretary of State for Social Services*, London, DHSS.

HALMOS, P. (1981) in HERAUD, B. *Training for Uncertainty*, London, Routledge and Kegan Paul.

HUNTINGTON, J. (1981) *Social Work and General Medical Practice*, London, George Allen and Unwin.

JOHNSON, T. (1972) *Professions and Power*, London, Macmillan.

JOURNALS (various issues): (i) *Almoner, The*; (ii) *Community Care*; (iii) *Medical Social Work*; (iv) *Nursing Mirror*; (v) *Nursing Times*; (vi) *Social Work*; (vii) *Social Work Today*.

LORENTZON, M. (1987) *Professional Status and Managerial Tasks — A Comparison of Nursing and Social Work in Contemporary Britain with Special Reference to Women's Work*, unpublished Ph.D. thesis, London School of Economics, University of London.

MORRIS, T. (1974) *The Marking of Cain*, an Inaugural Lecture, London School of Economics, University of London.

NEWMAN, G. (1983) *Just and Painful — A Case for the Corporal Punishment of Criminals*, London, Macmillan.

NURSES, MIDWIVES AND HEALTH VISITORS ACT (1979), London, HMSO.

PARRY, N. and PARRY, J. (1981) in HERAUD, B. *Training for Uncertainty*, London, RKP.

PARSLOE, P. / CCETSW (1983) Documents 20:1 and 20:2, London, CCETSW.

PARSONS, T. (1964) *Social Structure and Personality*, New York, Free Press.

PLATT, H. (1964) *A Reform of Nursing Education*, London, Royal College of Nursing.

POOR LAW CONFERENCE REPORTS (i) West Midlands (1884); (ii) South Wales (1901); (iii) Foreword to the 1903–1904 Volume; London, P. S. King and Sons.

PRINCE, J. (1984) 'Education for a Profession: Some Lessons from History', *International Journal of Nursing Studies*, **21**, 3, pp. 153–63.

PROCHASKA, F. K. (1980) *Women and Philanthropy in 19th Century England*, Oxford, Clarendon.

Project 2000 (1986) London, UKCC (United Kingdom Central Council for Nursing, Midwifery and Health Visiting).

ROSZAK, B. and ROSZAK, T. (1969) *Masculine/Feminine*, New York, Harper Torch Books.

RUSKIN, J. (1898) *Sesame and Lilies*, London, G. Allen Sunnyside, Orpington.

SALMON, B. (1966) *Report of the Committee on Senior Nursing Staff Structure*, London, HMSO.

SEEBOHM, F. (1968) *Report on Local and Allied Personal Social Services*, London, HMSO.

SMITH, F. B. (1982) *Florence Nightingale — Reputation and Power*, London, Croom Helm.

SPENDER, D. (1982) *Women of Ideas*, London, Ark Paperbacks.

STONE, L. (1980) in FISHER, E. *Woman's Creation — Sexual Evolution and the Shaping of Society*, London, Wildwood House.

TWINING, L. (1898) *Workhouses and Pauperism*, London, Methuen and Co.

WEBER, M. (1978) in RUNCIMAN, W. G. *Weber Selections in Translation*, Cambridge, CUP.

WOODHAM-SMITH, C. (1951) *Florence Nightingale, 1820–1910*, London, Fontana.

'WORKING FOR PATIENTS' (White Paper) (1989), London, Department of Health.

YOUNGHUSBAND, E. (1959) *Report of the Working Party on Social Workers in the Local Authority Health and Welfare Services*, London, HMSO.

YOUNGHUSBAND, E. (1978) *Social Work in Britain, 1950–1975, A Follow-up Study* Parts I and II, London, G. Allen and Unwin.

6
Social Work and Community Psychiatric Nursing

Michael Sheppard

Community psychiatric nursing (CPN) is a young profession, which has expanded and established itself largely in the last twenty years (Hunter, 1974, 1980). Given its relative youth, it is not surprising that research in this area is fairly sparse (Woof, 1987; Sladden, 1979; Parnell, 1978; Brooking, 1986). Although mental health social work is somewhat older, there is considerably less research in this area than, say, child care social work (Fisher *et al.*, 1984; Corney, 1984; Huxley *et al.*, 1987). There is still less literature comparing the work of both these professions (Woof, 1987; Woof *et al.*, 1988; Woof and Goldberg, 1988). In view of the long recognized needs of mentally ill people, the growth of knowledge in social psychiatry and the increasing emphasis on community care policies, both professions are assuming an increasingly important profile (Jones, 1988). It would be useful, therefore, to develop a conceptual framework upon which empirical developments may occur. This chapter will do this, and also summarize some results from a research programme which utilized this framework.

Social Work and CPN Role

It is useful first, however, to give a broad outline of the role of CPNs and mental health social workers. This is interesting because, to a considerable degree, they lay claim to the same 'occupational territory'; i.e., taking similar roles with similar client groups. Thus, Goldberg and Huxley (1980) comment that 'the community psychiatric nurse shares many skills with the social worker'.

Although social work has, compared with CPNs, a relatively long history, its modern form dates back to 1971 when major changes took place in the organization of social work. Prior to this social work was organized into different segments — child care officers, mental welfare officers, hospital social workers (almoners) and so on. Following the Seebohm Report, social workers became employed overwhelmingly in social service departments, rather than, as previously, in separate organizations. The notion of 'generic social work' — basically referring to common skills and knowledge applicable 'across the board' to social work problems — gained currency and was reflected in the literature in discussions about the 'common base' of social work practice (Bartlett, 1970; Barker, 1975, 1976). It also led to a tendency for social workers to take on a variety of different types of cases, which in an occupation with as great a diversity as social work led to accusations of 'deskilling' (Howe, 1980). More recently, social workers, when in area offices, have tended to develop interest in particular areas of practice, either on formal lines (where teams work in a specialized way) or informal lines (where social workers have a 'bias' in their caseloads towards particular client groups, e.g. child care or mental health). The initial effect of these developments, together with changes in the health service, was a reduction in specialist expertise in the mental health field. The Ottan Report (DHSS, 1974) protested that 'there is nothing in Seebohm to imply the wholesale abandonment of specialism in social work practice'. It is certainly the case that in more recent years specialist mental health social workers have become more widespread either based in mental health settings or by taking a specialist role in area teams.

The overall aim of social work, as prescribed by the Seebohm Report, was to provide a universally available community based and family oriented service. These broad areas were applicable to mental health social work in the same way as other aspects of social work. Traditionally social work in Britain has emphasized social casework — working mainly with individuals and families — as its primary mode of delivery (Davies, 1986). Applied to health settings the Ottan Report (DHSS, 1974) identified a variety of social work roles. These included assessment of psychosocial factors relevant, or contributing, to the health problems of the client; providing advice and input in relation to case management of social factors; provision of appropriate support for clients in the face of health difficulties, and contributing to an adequate care plan for those discharged from hospital. Within this frame, social workers were perceived to use skills in social assessment, social 'treatment' methods, use of resources and educational and consultancy work. The Barclay Report (NISW, 1982) has more recently extended the social work role. While recognizing the importance of direct individual and family work in relation to emotional and practical problems, it emphasized the development of social care networks: that is, providing networks of support in the community for those with emotional or practical problems. This represented a shift in emphasis (without abandoning more traditional roles) towards what was termed community social work.

Community psychiatric nursing services were first established in 1954 (Hunter, 1974). One obvious difference from social work is that CPNs were, from the start, employed in the health service. A rapid expansion in CPN services occurred from the early 1970s, when social workers were brought under social services departments. To a considerable degree this expansion occurred to fill the void left by social workers' move into a more generic form of service. Certainly, dissatisfaction has been expressed by psychiatric professions about the adequacy of mental health knowledge in the 'new' generic workers (Fisher, Newton and Sainsbury, 1984; Bean, 1980). It is perhaps not as easy to delineate, by comparison with social workers, the CPN role. There is no equivalent of either the Seebohm or Barclay Reports, and the development of CPN services has been sporadic, and their bases, modes of referral and ways of working have varied greatly. Skidmore and Friend (1984) have identified various types of setting: those which are hospital based; those based in primary care settings; those based jointly in hospital and primary care settings and those community based. The identification of role has been rather more haphazard than in social work, reflected in descriptions provided in the early CPN literature (Griffiths and Mangen, 1980). Like mental health social workers they have had a specialist interest in the mentally ill. Furthermore the available roles identified in Carr, Butterworth and Hodges (1980) resemble those of social workers. Broadly there has been an emphasis on continuity and extension of care and appropriate contact between hospital and community (Griffiths and Mangen, 1980). In more detail, CPNs are expected to carry out assessment of patients for nursing requirements, they are involved in therapeutic tasks related to counselling or more behavioural approaches; they act in a technical, clinical fashion, most noticeably in the provision of injections or individual care and advice in relation to health needs. Additionally CPN roles involve acting in terms of health education, informing people about risk in relation to mental disorder; acting as consultant in relation to other professionals, advising about the nature and appropriateness of psychiatric nursing care; and finally as managers organizing work priorities

There are clear similarities in the roles identified for CPNs and social workers — in particular the assessment, therapist, consultant and educator roles. The most noticeable difference is the clinical role adopted by CPNs (providing injections, etc.) and the community social work role identified in Barclay. One specialized role is that of the approved social worker, most highly profiled as applying in relation to assessments for compulsory admission (Sheppard, 1990).

Key Elements of Occupational Analysis

Having outlined the main roles of CPNs and social workers we may outline the framework for analyzing the work of these two occupations. Atkinson (1983) emphasizes the importance of influence provided by the transmission of knowledge on the behaviour of professions, and the reproduction of that behaviour in 'new' professionals. He advocates examining 'the relationship between education, practice and the organisation of occupational groups'. The knowledge and education of the profession will help develop characteristic traits in members of that profession. He emphasizes that knowledge is not simple, objective and uncontroversial but, through curriculm and values, is classified and combined in certain ways — it is a cultural imposition. This is significant because it suggests that the knowledge base of a profession will exercise a major influence on the way its members experience and define the world.

However, the *raison d'etre* for professional knowledge is its practice use: it is applied rather than pure in nature. The meaning attached to situations relates to the knowledge base and experience, and the balance of knowledge with the degree of emphasis on personal qualities or experience. This has relevance when comparing two or more professions. First, the discreteness of knowledge is significant: the more each profession has a knowledge base discrete to itself, the greater the expected difference in behaviour between the two professions. Second, however, this will also depend where on the spectrum of technicality–indeterminacy each professions's knowledge base is sited. The more indeterminate it is, the less the knowledge base differences will matter. Third, where close contacts exist between two professions we would expect shared experience and negotiation of meanings would lead to learning and increased similarities in behaviour (depending of course on the extent of knowledge indeterminacy).

At the base of our framework we have emphasized the place of knowledge in the understanding of the way a profession will attach meaning to, or interpret, situations. The framework will be divided as follows:

1 Knowledge orientation
2 Practice orientation
3 Defining the patient or client
4 Context of intervention
5 Contexts specific to mental health
6 Direct and indirect work
7 Duration of intervention

The analysis will conceptualize CPNs and mental health social workers as branches of their professions, i.e. emphasizing one to be a nurse and the other a social worker.

Knowledge Orientation

Social work has, for some considerable time, emphasized its social science knowledge base (Leonard, 1975; Bartlett, 1970). This social science emphasis produces predefined categories — stigma, class, socialization, attachment, etc. — which provide a means for interpreting situations through a range of alternative explanations. Hence child battering may occur through stress, failure of attachment, poverty, cycle of abuse and so on (Sheppard, 1982). They provide *reasons* or *causes* for what is occurring, thus making clients' actions meaningful. They provide a means for interpreting behaviour.

However, there is no unified professional view of the place of social science knowledge — an illustration of professional segmentation. Some — although a small minority — have sought to marginalize social science. Davies (1986) suggests that social science — and sociology in particular — has done little to improve practice, while Howe (1980) argues that social science is riven by such great paradigmatic and theoretical disputes as to make it difficult to develop a knowledge base or apply it with any effectiveness. Despite Davies' criticisms, and although debate exists about *how* it should be applied, social science remains the dominant knowledge base for social work. Indeed, Hardiker (1981) maintains it is indispensable, drawing on research to demonstrate that it makes the difference between adequate practice and possible disasters.

The presentation of the CPN knowledge base is different in a number of respects. Reflecting professional role, knowledge focuses specifically on mental health. Although there is some variation (Davis, 1986; Kalkman and Davis, 1974) this is generally organized in terms of models or psychiatric ideologies. Two reasons for their significance are presented: constructing a model of mental illness allows us to see its nature, causation and effects (Mitchell, 1974); and they allow nurses to function rationally and evaluate their effectiveness (Stuart and Sundeen, 1983). The use of models is allied to the general advocacy of eclecticism. It is seen as a means of overcoming the 'limitations' and 'simplifications' of theory, and the belief that there is no 'right way' to approach problems (Lancaster, 1980). Neither eclecticism nor the choice of model is generally seen as problematic — choice may be based on the nurse's personal preference, provided it is explicit (Burgess, 1985). Although some social workers also advocate eclecticism (Pincus and Minahan, 1975; Whittaker, 1974), they appear more aware of inherent inconsistencies, the threat to developing a consistent knowledge base and the need for rigorous criteria to choose between models. 'The nursing literature', writes Sladden, 'does not waste time over the conceptual problems of the eclectic approach' (Sladden, 1979). The delineation of models reflects an awareness of their interest to psychiatry as a whole (Siegler and Osmond, 1966; Strauss *et al.*, 1964; Tyrer and Steinberg, 1987). Model construction, however, varies between different authors. The core division, identifying medical, social and psychological models, is presented by Mitchell (1974). The medical model (Burgess calls this 'biologic') presents psychiatric disorder like any other involving a pathological lesion and disturbed function which is resolved physiologically (e.g. by drugs). Others add a characteristic process of examination, diagnosis, treatment and prognosis (Carr *et al.*, 1980; Stuart and Sundeen, 1983). Mitchell suggests the social model focuses on individuals' failure to function in groups, while others emphasize the causal significance of social environment and conditions, additionally emphasizing that mental illness is culturally defined (Stuart and Sundeen, 1983). The third model is psychological, which is presented as behavioural disturbance or distress due to powerful psychological forces, resolved only by therapy confronting the intra-psychic conflicts. However, further distinctions exist. Additional divisions exist between psychoanalytic and behavioural or cognitive behavioural models (Burgess, 1985; Stuart and Sundeen, 1983), and 'Third Force' psychology emphasizing people's potential for personal growth. Stuart and Sundeen (1983) present two further models, existential and interpersonal, emphasizing the importance of relations *between* people. A 'community orientation', loosely defined as an ideology focusing on those needing help but unwilling or unable to seek it, is identified by Carr *et al.* (1980) (cf. Baker and Schulberg, 1967). Finally Davey (1984) identifies an anti-psychiatry perspective (better called perspectives) broadly denying the validity of an illness label for those suffering psychiatric problems. Overall, although models may be helpful, the CPN is confronted by a great, perhaps bewildering, variety of alternatives and no consensus about divisions between them.

Practice Orientation: Judgment and Experience

The limited nature of social science knowledge concomitantly increases the importance of judgment and experience, well recognized in social work. Indeed, those who emphasize social work as 'art' rather than 'technique' stress this most strongly. What is important in the process of social work, and what is effective in achieving its ends, they argue, is not some technical expertise, but the quality of the person of the helper (Jordan, 1979; Keith-Lucas, 1972). While some people help, other people may impede progress. To a considerable degree this emphasizes the understanding of others by social workers. This involves using abilities which most of us possess, but the social worker — to be any good — should develop to an advanced level. 'The worker knows about the client's meaning because the worker's own ''human nature'' tells him what it is to experience . . . mental or emotional states and can sensitively extrapolate from them' (England, 1986). Additionally, their work leads to contact with problems to a far greater degree than normal social life, and their work involves focusing on these problems. Hence practice experience allows them to refine their understanding and responses to these problems, thus providing a legitimate 'knowledge base' in itself.

The issue of judgment is significant for nursing as a whole and CPNs in particular, though not all are agreed. Neuman (1980) and Johnson (1980) both emphasize the technical expertise derived from their models. Orem (1980) however, recognizes the importance of particular techniques but emphasizes the individual patient and correct nursing judgments. Most significant for good judgment, she suggests, is the nurse's experience, but other factors such as innate ability, life experience, personality and style of thinking are also important. Rogers (1970) also sees a relationship between the technical aspects of knowledge and the more creative, individualized, and to a considerable degree experience based use of judgment in applying that knowledge.

It is, then, as with social work, the limitations of knowledge when applied to practice which leave experience and judgment a vital place in practice. Lack of experience and good judgment can be inimicable to good (or even minimally adequate) practice. In theoretical terms, judgment and experience are significant because they limit the effect on behaviour of knowledge approaches discrete to each profession. Of course, experience is not somehow divorced from theory — implicitly or explicitly used to give situations meaning. However, the more important experience is, the more scope exists for creative understanding and responses to problems on the part of individual practitioners. Indeed, where frequent contact occurs, this may well encourage 'seepage' of concepts and theories from one discipline to another.

Defining the Client or Patient

Both social workers and CPNs define clients with meanings particular to their profession: either in terms of problems or needs. Social workers' concern is with *psychosocial* problems or needs (Haines, 1975; Roberts and Nee, 1970). Reid (1978) distinguishes between *acknowledged* problems — problems clients consider themselves to have — and *attributed* problems — problems attributed by others, in this case social workers, to clients. Furthermore, fundamental disagreements exist about problem definition. What does or does not constitute a social problem depends upon the social processes by which it becomes a matter of concern, as well as theoretical assumptions underlying them (Rubington and Weinberg, 1977). Social work definitions of problems possess implicit standards influenced greatly by their position in social service departments (Howe, 1979).

Need definitions also possess an ideological dimension. Hardiker (1981; cf. Davies, 1982) argues that: 'The social worker's brief in welfare states is to identify and meet personal need and find acceptable ways of representing deviants to the rest of society'. Their freedom to define need, however, she considers is limited by structural boundaries provided by their agency. Smith and Harris (1972), like other authors, argue that social workers adopt ideologies of need based on perceptions of unit of need, cause of need and assessor of need. Rees (1978) indicates these ideologies are related closely to perceptions of moral character, while Hardiker (1977) suggests they are keys to understanding central issues of punishment/freewill and treatment/ determinism, and that interpretations of need are made through frameworks originating from psychological or sociological knowledge.

Nursing differs form social work in its emphasis on health. Their bio-psychosocial orientation is more ambitious than that of social work, which emphasizes only the psychosocial (Kim, 1983; Chrisman and Fowler, 1980; Pearson and Vaughn, 1984; Roper *et al.*, 1980; Kyes and Hofling, 1980). Kim (1983) argues that problem or need definition is critical for nursing diagnosis, providing a means for conceptualizing the client in terms of the concerns of nursing. This is just as true for CPNs: Simmons and Brooker (1986) state that 'true mental health requires basic needs are met'. However, when need is explored more deeply, there is little reference to its ideological component. Maslow's hierarchy of need — which is, like other need definitions, ideological — is particularly influential (Maslow, 1970). This identifies a hierarchy of need, with five levels from basic physiological needs through more 'advanced' needs up to self actualization. These are ordered in priority: it is only when the lower needs are satisfied that motivation is established to seek fulfilment of higher level needs.

Nursing is also conceived in terms of problems. Rambo (1984) indeed recognizes the relevance of both need and problem definition, but suggests the superiority of the latter by linking it with scientificity. 'The nursing process', she writes, 'as a method of problem solving represents a scientific avenue of nursing care'. Barker (1985) likewise prefers problem identification to (medical) diagnosis in psychiatric nursing. 'The common denominator', he suggests, 'is the search for and ultimate detection of, problems . . . Aspects of a person's performance and presentation which might be ignored or overlooked in [medical] diagnosis will be caught under this broader frame of reference.' Problem definition in nursing reflects nursing's concern with the biopsychosocial aspects of the human condition. Stevens (1979), for example, lists five conditions: experientail states, physiological deviations, problematic behaviour, altered relationships and reactions of others. However, problem identification is to some degree theory related — hence different approaches will emphasize different aspects (Roy and Roberts, 1981; Orem, 1980).

However, what is required is a problem classification which is framed in terms of meanings appropriate to CPNs (and social workers) and which may be applied across different models (Kim, 1983). Kim suggests problem identification requires three elements: a problem label, a definition of causal elements, and a description of the characteristics of the phenomenon, interestingly close to that advocated by Huntington (1981) for social work.

Context of Intervention

The context of social work practice reflects its psychosocial orientation — the 'knowledge space' occupied by the profession — and the related intervention modes. Social work possesses theoretical diversity and some conflicting assumptions. Practice is rarely characterized by explicit use of theory, but when examined closely, theoretical constructs provide an implicit though critical context for practice. Curnock and Hardiker (1979) have shown that good practice requires theory, without which mistakes would be made. It necessarily involves flexible and imaginative use of such theory. However, because of this theoretical diversity, it is difficult to characterize social work in terms of a particular approach: it is best reflected in the pragmatic use of different contexts for intervention rather than specific methods which may be adopted. Analysis based on a specific method would not reflect the known, and diverse, use of theory in practice.

Recent theoretical developments suggest four stages. The basic division is between interpersonal intervention, largely but not exclusively concerned with clients, and environmental intervention, involving individuals and systems within the social structure in the process of providing services to the client (Haines, 1975). This configuration, classically presented by Hollis (1964), was 'person in situation': the person, his situation and the interaction between them. She referred to 'internal' and 'external' pressure to signify forces within the individual and the environment. Drawing on psychoanalytic and sociological concepts, intervention involved addressing both internal psychological conflicts and 'life pressures' such as economic deprivation, poor housing and educational disadvantage.

Bartlett's (1970) concern with social work's overemphasis on the client's immediate circumstances led to her conception of 'intervention repertoire', involving the use of a variety of approaches as appropriate. Hence the practitioner may involve themselves with the client, encourage groups, develop social supports and act for change within the community. Work could be both proactive and reactive.

Unitary models attempted to provide a conceptual schema for the repertoire, moving beyond a 'dichotomous view' of people and environment, to a focus on linkages between people and resource systems (Pincus and Minahan, 1975). This system approach meant the issue was not: 'who has the problem, but how the elements of the situation . . . are interacting to frustrate people coping with their tasks'. The ecological perspective has much in common with unitary models. However, it goes one stage further by identifying 'levels' of context. Whittaker and Garbarino (1983) developed a four-fold distinction based on concepts of social networks and support. To a considerable degree this provides a theoretical base for community social work developments (NISW, 1982). Microsystems represent the immediate social networks of individuals — their family, school, immediate workplace and so on. Mesosystems are the relationships *between* these microsystems (e.g. relations between home, school and work related groups). Exosystems are situations that affect a person's development, but in which the person does not play a direct role. Macrosystems are ideological and cultural expectations in a society: they reflect shared beliefs creating behavioural patterns (e.g. how cultures define and respond to dependency, how political ideologies allocate resources between public and private agencies and different groups). Whittaker (1974) calls work using this ecological approach 'social treatment'. He defines five major roles (Whittaker, 1986):

1 Treatment agent
2 Teacher/counsellor
3 Broker of services or resources
4 Advocate
5 Network/systems consultant

Each of these represent role clusters — ways of working or responsibilities the professional may assume according to the circumstances of the case — and may operate in different and overlapping contexts

Woof (1987) suggests community psychiatric nursing is characterized by the lack of a theoretical base: 'neither psychiatric nurses or CPNs have developed a common set of principles or an organised set of professional values . . . integral . . . for decision making skills'. However, models exist in the wider realm of nursing as a whole. In this respect it resembles social work — possessing models which are, on the whole, general to the profession but not specifice to psychiatry. Kim (1983) classifies nursing in terms of its domain. Using Kim, we can distinguish two arenas in the *domain* of nursing — the phenomena with which it is concerned — that focusing on the patient and that focusing on the environment. Beyond Kim's typology, however, we can distinguish the *context* of nursing — the phenomena on which it will act — from its domain. This likewise can be divided between client and environment.

Although a variety of different approaches are available — activities of living, interpersonal, total person, behavioural systems and so on — two broad factors are consistent to these models. First, nursing concerns itself with biopsychosocial factors affecting health. This is both all-embracing in terms of the human condition and more ambitious than the more limited psychosocial concerns of social work. Second, while the *domains* of interest of nursing frequently encompass biopsychosocial aspects of both patient and environment, the *context* of intervention invariably focuses primarily on the patient.

This can, at times, appear as a puzzling disjunction between domains relevant to health, such as social factors which suggest the need for environmental intervention, and the specific intervention focus on the patient. This may be related to perceptions of the appropriate role of the nurse, which would lead to the development of role appropriate models for practice. This individualism is consistent with some models emphasizing nurse–patient interaction. King's (1981) theory of goal attainment emphasizes interactional elements — particularly 'nurse–client interactions that lead to achievement of goals'. She is quite explicit: although the domains of concern for nursing are personal, interpersonal and social systems, and health problems may be caused by environmental stress, the main focus for action is the nurse–patient dyad.

Others claim domains which are equally comprehensive, without being explicit, as King is, about the narrower focus for intervention. Rogers' (1970) concept of unitary man accepts only the interconnectedness, *in reality*, of environmental and human elements, although conceding the possibility of distinguishing *conceptually* between the two. Johnson's model (Johnson, 1980; Grubb, 1980) recognizes physical, psychological and social elements, and expresses interest in the domains of both client and environment. Grubb (1980) lists a number of relevant environmental variables, yet: 'the predominant focus of nursing is on the person who is ill or threatened with illness'. Roy also recognizes both personal and environmental variables, with physiological, self concept, role function and interdependence elements (Roy and Roberts, 1981). She, however emphasizes the need for individual adaptation to the environment whether involving biophysical or social elements. This, of course, begs the question: just how adequate for health is the environment to which the patient must adapt?

This disjunction between domain and context is well illustrated by Rambo's (1984) explication of Roy's model. She clearly recognizes many American black people's health is affected by structural disadvantage, involving segregation, discrimination and poverty. She also recognizes these can affect the patient's health and performance, causing maladaptive behaviour, with which the nurse is legitimately concerned. Yet the nurse should only work with the patient to: 'attempt ot bring *their* [my italics] maladaptive behaviour within the normal or adaptive range'. Some writers do recognize approaches beyond the individual, although they are more tentative and lack the alternatives available to social work. Kim (1983) differentiates between the client–nurse system, involving nurse–patient interaction, and the nurse system, largely excluding the patient, but does little more. Pepleau, whose interest is primarily in a therapeutic inter-personal process, does advocate involvement in health care planning and social policy issues (Pepleau, 1952, 1980). However, between individual work and social policy issues, she has little on work with patients in an environmental context. Neuman (1982) goes further in this direction. She recognizes nurses' claim to be concerned with phenomena relating to both client and environment. She identifies stressors originating in intrapersonal, interpersonal and extrapersonal areas. Additionally, however, she suggests preventive care and health education programmes, and that nurses should help 'individuals, families and groups' attain a maximum level of wellness (Neuman, 1980). Chapman (1985) suggests this model is useful applied not just to individuals but also communities.

This dominant individualist focus — contrasting with detailed theoretical developments beyond individual clients in social work — is significant because, as Kim (1983) suggests, the focus provides a 'space' within which knowledge and skills may develop. A dominant individualism militates against the inclusion of skills oriented to the environment in the nurses' repertoire.

Contexts Specific to Mental Health

Social work approaches to mental health problems largely entail the application of their broader professional skills to the more specific area of mental health. As with other areas of work such as child care, they limit their concern — wide enough in itself — to the psychosocial, perceived to complement the more biophysical medical orientation of psychiatrists. This approach is supported by social psychiatry research which has emphasized the interconnection between those very personal and environmental factors on which social work skills concentrate (Cochrane, 1983; Miles, 1987). Much of the social work knowledge development specific to psychiatry involves identification and recognition of mental disorders, core — in more detail — to psychiatric nurse training, examining this in terms of the social process, context and prognosis of mental illness (Hodson, 1982; Munro and McCulloch, 1969; Butler and Pritchard, 1983). In recent years, Approved Social Work training has emphasized the legal context as well as symptom recognition plus specific skills in case material analysis (CCETSW, 1986).

The theoretical limits of nursing as a whole clearly disadvantage CPNs interested in placing patients within a broader environmental context. Indeed, the community rather than institutional hospital perspective has led to an emphasis on individualized care of the patient (Carr *et al.*, 1980; Ward, 1985). Some attempts to incorporate a psychosocial dimension have not transcended this individualism Hence Barry (1984), developing Roy's adaptation model, focuses on the patient, emphasizing psychological rather than social variables. Likewise, Barker (1985) emphasizes a 'person centred approach' designed to identify what is significant for 'this particular patient' who is 'a unique person'.

In the face of theoretical limitations, CPNs have, to a considerable degree, taken refuge in skills information, pragmatically chosen on the basis of professional need (Marram, 1973; Looms and Horsely, 1974). This is largely 'borrowed' knowledge, generated within other disciplines, but apparently useful to CPNs. In this respect, approaches to social skills, and particularly behaviourism have taken on some signficance (Roach and Farley, 1986; Marks *et al.*, 1977; Barker, 1982; Pope, 1986; Hargie and McCarton, 1986). Given the psychological orientation, the focus tends primarily to be on the individual, although there is a greater interest in their immediate interactional context, as with behavioural approaches. Likewise Pope (1986) discusses the use of family skills training with schizophrenic patients' families who express high levels of emotion.

A potentially wider context is provided by an ecological approach (Lancaster, 1980) emphasizing the 'dynamic interaction between the patient's internal environment and the multiple external environments'. These are linked by a systems approach, but there is little theoretical development, such as different types and levels of environmental intervention. Rather, there are hints of relevant factors such as familial or social systems linkages, which are not fully developed. The exploration of the context of social environment has been rather too brief for detailed skills of development (Carr *et al.*, 1980). Simmons and Brooker (1986) have been boldest in this respect, examining in some detail social factors in the family and wider society. Their analysis is stimulating, suggesting wider possible contexts for intervention, but ultimately limited in detail about the ways to work in these wider social contexts.

Overall, then, while nursing does possess a theoretical base, CPNs may be viewed as struggling to free themselves from its limits. They have taken a few tentative steps without developing a consistent theoretical base beyond individualism.

Direct and Indirect Work

The client/enviroment distinction relevant to both social work and nursing may be related to direct and indirect work. This is a distinction extensively used in social work as a means of delineating the locus of intervention (Specht and Vickery, 1978; Whittaker, 1974; Haines, 1975; Whittaker and Garbarino, 1983). In our framework it is significant because it indicates the worker's approach to particular problems, hence linking problem type with locus of intervention. Whittaker (1974) adopts the most frequently used definitions. Direct work is 'what the worker does directly in their face to face encounter'. Indirect helping 'refers to all activities that the worker undertakes on behalf of the client to further mutually agreed upon goals', i.e. work with others designed to influence the client's behaviour and/or circumstances.

Duration of Intervention

The final element is the duration of intervention. Extended work is associated with three general influences. Psychoanalysis has influenced significantly the knowledge base of social work. With its emphasis on in-depth analysis of underlying psychological problems, and development of 'insight' (a term used by social workers differently from psychoanalysts) it has a tendency towards lengthy intervention (Yelloly, 1980; Hollis, 1964).

Others regard the 'relationship' as crucial. By valuing relationships for their own sake, and where the goal is presented as self realization or self-fulfilment, importance is implicitly attached to extended intervention (Keith-Lucas, 1972; Jordan, 1979). Although an end in itself, the relationship is also seen as the most effective means of promoting change (Truax and Carkhuff, 1967). A third associated element is a generalized 'supportive' orientation of some social workers. In mental health work, the professional role becomes a form of 'unlimited supportive friendship' in jeopardy (Fisher *et al.*, 1984). Extended intervention may be long term by design, but tends instead to be 'open ended' rather than time limited. It may be of low or high intensity or anywhere between (in number of interviews per time period).

Brief intervention is associated with task centred and crisis intervention while some behavioural work can also be time limited (Reid, 1978; Rappaport, 1970; Sheldon, 1982, 1983). Crisis intervention emphasizes the therapeutic potential of work over a relatively short crisis period (Rappaport, 1970). During this period the client is in a state of disequilibrium, when normal problem solving techniques are ineffective. However, there are natural processes of growth and development which, during this time, the worker may help mobilize in the client. Key characteristics of this approach are that it is both goal oriented and time limited, in this respect similar to task centred work. These also emphasize exactitude in formulating problems, methods to deal with them, and evaluation of outcome. Task centred work is more widely applicable, not limited to states or crisis. Rather than emphasizing in-depth work (or 'underlying conditions'), task centred work directs change efforts at *manifest* problems of interpersonal conflict — role performance and the like — working on the 'here and now'.

Although there is an element of expediency in advocating brief intervention (given limited resources) supporters argue it is no less effective than extended work (Reid, 1978). Some intervention is unintentionally brief because clients discontinue contact, but debates on duration reflect basic differences in philosophies of practice.

Comments

Although neither social work nor CPN is rigidly demarked by approaches discrete to each profession, they are characterized by significant differences of emphasis. Hence neither adopts an inflexible collection code, but each is characterized by different elements (and degrees) of integration. Thus the biopsychosocial CPN orientation adopts models from wider realms of knowledge, but this is far from systematic, lacking criteria for integration. Problems of eclecticism arise which are not confronted. Social work, with a less ambitious psychosocial orientation, has considered issues of integration within its narrower social science framework (Sheldon, 1978; Sheppard, 1984; Stevenson, 1971; Whittaker and Garbarino, 1985).

Both professions, furthermore, recognize a significant degree of indetermination; hence the importance of judgment. When combined with paradigmatic and knowledge realm diversity, this indeterminacy encourages segmentation within these professions, with individuals or groups committed to different approaches. There is, furthermore, some overlap between these professions. Hence the uncertainty of the social science foundations of social work is reflected in the variety of available mental health models; significance is ascribed by both professions to judgment; both claim an interest in the psychosocial (though CPNs are also interested in the 'bio'); and both borrow knowledge from other disciplines, although unlike CPNs, social workers have also generated their own knowledge (e.g. task centred, problem solving).

However, significant differences exist. Some issues of relevance to both professions, such as the duration of intervention, have been considered in detail only by social work. CPN's theoretical base is more individualistic and far less well developed than that of social work. At the same time CPNs claim a domain — biopsychosocial — far wider than that of social work. To a considerable degree this means they raise problems — such as the social disadvantage–illness relationship — with which their theory (or model) does not equip them to deal. Perhaps harshly we might say that CPNs make greater claims than social workers but have less ability to 'deliver the goods'.

The conceptual framework is important also because it can generate hypotheses, or at least identify issues, using meanings appropriate to both professions to be examined in comparative research. Questions arise about the definition of clients, context of intervention, knowledge orientation, duration of intervention and so on which can be examined in practice. These revolve around the broad issue raised by Atkinson: the influence of the transmission of knowledge on the behaviour of professional groups. This is no purely academic issue: it has major practice implications, contributing to our understanding both of the appropriate education for these professions and also the most appropriate mode of service delivery (and who is best suited to provide it).

Research Findings

Research has been undertaken enabling the examination of social work and CPN practice in the light of the framework outlined. It involved two teams, one of mental health social workers and the other of CPNs. These were based in the same setting, a mental health advice centre, facilitating comparison because they had available the same range of clientele (referred to the centre).

The results for brief intervention, generally lasting a week or less, showed few differences. Indeed the practice of the two occupations was notable for the similarities rather than the differences. Major differences, however, were identified in relation to extended intervention which indicate that social workers and CPNs took on entirely different roles. Indeed the style of intervention adopted suggests, far from these occupations being interchangeable in terms of community mental health work, that the service to clients would vary greatly according to which profession was allocated the case.

The differences confirm, to a considerable degree, expectations arising from the examination of occupational socialization and discourse. Social workers define their clients primarily in terms of social problems, whereas mental health case definitions received a higher profile amongst CPNs. Social workers, according to the main indicators — role, context and indirect work — operated in a wider community context than CPNs. Social workers acted as advocate or resource mobilizers, worked with outside agencies and professionals, and tackled more practical, emotional and relationship problems indirectly to a far greater extent than CPNs. Indeed, in terms of active use of community resources and agencies, CPN work appears to have been negligible. Where outside agencies were involved CPNs had a particularly strong health orientation although this was noticeable also in the case of social workers. Indeed where agencies and professionals were involved CPNs appeared to have shown a very strong reliance on contact with doctors.

The social work task, furthermore, seems to have been more complex. Social workers identified significantly more severe problems, and had significantly more severe multi-problem clients. Social workers undertook more activities per client — they actually 'did more' in client management. Indeed there was a generally narrower range to CPNs' work: they had a narrower range of problems, smaller repertoire of roles, and undertook fewer activities. The number of interviews and duration of intervention undertaken by social workers was greater than CPNs. Indeed, not only was intervention on the whole longer, the *intensity* of intervention was greater by social workers.

Despite this, CPNs rated themslves, on the whole, to be more helpful to clients than social workers. This is particularly interesting, for it suggests an optimistic view of outcome. Such an optimistic view might leave them less inclined critically to assess or evaluate their work, on the basis that it was on the whole successful (alternatively social workers, with a less optimistic view and perhaps more demanding of themselves, may be more self critical). Social workers, furthermore, were more prepared to accept cases in which, on the evidence of the index of helpfulness, they considered themselves less likely to be helpful.

Overall, therefore, the similarities identified with brief intervention appear very much related to the brevity of intervention. This may be because its brevity did not allow workers to demonstrate a wider range of skills or approaches — there simply was not enough time. Alternatively the range of skills required for brief intervention may have been narrower, and fitted comfortably into the approaches of both CPNs and social workers. However, and this is important for professional image, this may indicate that others may perceive the CPN and social work roles to be interchangeable while this is not, in fact, so. Outside professionals would have a relatively limited contact with CPNs and social workers, and its brevity may have the effect of making the work of these two occupations appear similar.

There is some suggestion that CPNs were more rigid in their approaches, arising from narrower skills rather than theory emphasis. Hence their narrower range of work was matched by fewer activities and limited repertoire of roles. Theoretical approaches which had a broader community orientation and that linked skills which could be used in different community contexts may have widened the approaches they made. This conclusion is very much in line with evidence from the literature on nursing models.

Examination of extended intervention, therefore, suggests that although they do have a role of their own, CPNs are not well positioned to take over the traditional social work role. This is particularly interesting because of the close collaboration in much of their work (in the same agency) between CPNs and social workers. It may be that this collaboration has sufficient impact to affect practice over a relatively short period of time. However, individual responsibility over a longer period of time clearly demonstrates differences. If 'seepage' of ideas did occur they did not have sufficient impact to make differences insignificant. Indeed, the results, to a considerable degree, are in line with expectations arising from socialization.

Note

1. Mental health models and social science reflect the terms of discourse for social work and CPN knowledge. This does not prevent social workers from considering mental health models (much discussed by social scientists) or CPNs from considering social science influences on mental health models.

References

ATKINSON, P. (1977) 'The reproduction of professional knowledge', in DINGWALL, R., HEATH, C., REID, M. and STACEY, M. (Eds) *Health Care and Health Knowledge*, London, Croom Helm.

ATKINSON, P. (1983) 'The Reproduction of the Professional Community', in DINGWALL, R. and LEWIS, P. (Eds) *The Sociology of the Professions: Lawyers, Doctors and Others*, London, Macmillan.

BAKER, F. and SCHULBERG, E. (1967) 'The development of a community mental health ideology scale', *Community Mental Health Journal*, 3, pp. 216–51.

BARKER, P.J. (1982) *Behavioural Therapy Nursing*, London, Croom Helm.

BARKER, P.J. (1985) *Patient Assessment in Psychiatric Nursing*, London, Croom Helm.

BARKER, R. (1975) 'Towards generic social work practice: a review and some innovations', *British Journal of Social Work*, 5, 2, pp. 193–215.

BARKER, R. (1976) 'The multi role practitioner in the generic orientation to social work practice', *British Journal of Social Work*, 6, 3, pp. 327–51.

BARRY, P.D. (1984) *Psychosocial Nursing Assessment and Instruction*, London, J.P.L. Lipincott.

BARTLETT, H. (1970) *The Common Base of Social Work Practice*, Washington, DC, National Association of Social Workers.

BEAN, P. (1980) *Compulsory Admissions to Mental Hospitals*, London, Routledge and Kegan Paul.

BERNSTEIN, B. (1971) 'On the Classification and Framing of Educational Knowledge', in YOUNG, M.F.D. (Ed.) *Knowledge and Control: New Directions for the Sociology of Education*, London, Collier Macmillan.

BERNSTEIN, B. (1975) *Class, Codes and Control. Volume 3. Towards a Theory of Educational Transmissions*, London, Routledge and Kegan Paul.

BROOKING, J. (Ed.) (1986) *Psychiatric Nursing Research*, New York, McGraw Hill.

BUCHER, R. and STRAUSS, A. (1966) 'Professions in Process', *American Journal of Sociology*, 66, pp. 325–34.

BURGESS, A.W. (1985) *Psychiatric Nursing in the Hospital and Community*, Englewood Cliffs, N.J., Prentice Hall.

BURRELL, G. and MORGAN, G. (1979) *Sociological Paradigms and Organisational Analysis* London, Heinemann.

BUTLER, A. and PRITCHARD, C. (1983) *Social Work and Mental Illness*, London, Macmillan.

CARR, P.J., BUTTERWORTH, C.A. and HODGES, B.E. (1980) *Community Psychiatric Nursing*, London, Churchill Livingstone.

C.C.E.T.S.W. (1986) *Paper 19·17 Approved Social Workers' Report of the CCETSW Examinations Board*, London, C.C.E.T.S.W.

CHAPMAN, C.M. (1985) *Theory of Nursing: Practical Application*, London, Harper and Row.

CHRISMAN, M. and FOWLER, M. (1980) 'The systems change model for nursing practice', in RIEHL, J. P. and ROY, C. (Eds) *Conceptual Models for Nursing Practice,* 2nd. ed., London, Prentice Hall.

COCHRANE, R. (1983) *The Social Creation of Mental Illness,* Hong Kong, Longmans.

CORNEY, R. (1984) *The Effectiveness of Attached Social Workers in the Management of Depressed Female Patients in General Practice,* London, Cambridge University Press.

COROB, A. (1987) *Working with Depressed Women: A Feminist Approach,* Aldershot, Gower.

CURNOCK, K. and HARDIKER, P. (1979) *Towards Practice Theory Skills and Methods in Social Assessment,* London, Routledge and Kegan Paul.

DAVEY, P. T. (1984) *Theory and Practice of Psychiatric Care,* London, Hodder and Stoughton.

DAVIES, M. (1974) 'The Current State of Social Work Research', *British Journal of Social Work,* 4, pp. 281–305.

DAVIES, M. (1982) 'A Comment on Heart or Head', *Issues in Social Work Education,* 2, 1, pp. 57–60.

DAVIES, M. (1986) *The Essential Social Worker,* 2nd ed., Aldershot, Gower.

DAVIS B. (1986) 'A Review of Recent Research in Psychiatric Nursing', in BROOKING, J. (Ed.) *Psychiatric Nursing Research,* Chichester, John Wiley and Son.

DEPARTMENT OF HEALTH AND SOCIAL SECURITY (1974) *Social Work Support for the Health Service: Report of Working Party* (Ottan Report), London, HMSO.

ENGLAND, H. (1986) *Social Work as Art,* London, George Allen and Unwin.

FISHER, M., NEWTON, C. and SAINSBURY, E. (1984) *Mental Health Social Work Observed,* London, George Allen and Unwin

FREIDSON, E. (1970) *The Profession of Medicine,* New York, Harper and Row.

GOLDBERG, D. and HUXLEY, P. (1980) *Mental Illness in the Community,* London, Tavistock.

GRIFFITH, J. H. and MANGEN, S. P. (1980) 'Community Psychiatric Nursing: A literature review', *International Journal of Nursing Studies,* 17, pp. 197–210.

GRUBB, J. (1980) 'An Interpretation of the Johnson Behavioural System Model for Nursing Practice', in REIHL, J. P. and ROY, C. (Eds) *Conceptual Models for Nursing Practice,* 2nd ed., London, Prentice Hall.

HAINES, J. (1975) *Skills and Methods in Social Work,* London, Constable.

HARDIKER, P. (1977) 'Social Work Ideologies in the Probation Service', *British Journal of Social Work,* 7, pp. 131–54.

HARDIKER, P. (1981) 'Heart or Head. The Function and Role of Knowledge in Social Work', *Issues in Social Work Education,* 2, 1, pp. 85–112.

HARGIE, O. and MCCARTON, P. (1986) *Social Skills Training and Psychiatric Nursing,* London, Croom Helm.

HARRE, R. (1970) *The Principles of Scientific Thinking,* London, Macmillan.

HENDERSON, V. (1964) *Basic Principles of Nursing Care,* Geneva, International Council of Nurses.

HOGHUGHI, M. (1980) 'Social Work in a Bind', *Community Care,* 3 November, pp. 17–23.

HOLLIS, R. (1964) *Casework: A Psychosocial Therapy,* London, Columbia University Press.

HOWE, D. (1979) 'Agency Function and Social Work Principles', *British Journal of Social Work,* 9, pp. 29–48.

HOWE, D. (1980) 'Inflated States and Empty Theories in Social Work', *British Journal of Social Work,* 10, pp. 317–40.

HODSON, B. (1982) *Social Work with Psychiatric Patients,* London, Macmillan.

HUNTER, P. (1974) 'Community Psychiatric Nursing in Britain: an historical review', *International Journal of Nursing Studies,* 11, pp. 223–33.

HUNTER. P. (1980) 'Social Work and Community Psychiatric Nursing — A Review', *International Journal of Nursing Studies,* 17, pp. 131–9.

HUNTINGTON, J. (1981) *Social Work and General Medical Practice. Collaboration or Conflict,* London, George Allen and Unwin.

HUXLEY, P., KORER, J. and TOLLEY, S. (1987) 'The Psychiatric "Caseness" of Clients Referred to an Urban Social Services Department', *British Journal of Social Work,* 17, pp. 507–20.

JAMOUS, H. and PELOILLE, B. (1970) 'Professions or self perpetuating systems? Changes in the French University-Hospital System', in JACKSON, J. A. (Ed.) *Professions and Socialisation,* Cambridge, Cambridge University Press.

JOHNSON, D. (1980) 'The Behavioural Systems Model' in REIHL, J. P. and ROY, C. (Eds) *Conceptual Models for Nursing,* 2nd ed., London, Prentice Hall.

JONES, K. (1988) *Experience in Mental Health: Community Care and Social Policy,* London, Sage.

JORDAN, W. (1979) *Helping in Social Work,* London, Routledge and Kegan Paul.

KALKMAN, M. and DAVIS, A. (Eds) (1974) *Dimensions of Mental Health — Psychiatric Nursing,* New York, McGraw Hill.

KEAT, R. and URRY, J. (1982) *Social Theory as Science,* 2nd ed., London, Routledge and Kegan Paul.

KEITH-LUCAS, A. (1972) *Giving and Taking Help,* Chapel Hill, University of North Carolina Press.

KIM, H. S. (1983) *The Nature of Theoretical Thinking in Nursing,* London, Prentice Hall.

KING, I. M. (1981) *A Theory for Nursing,* London, John Wiley.

KYES, J. and HOFLING, C. (1980) *Basic Psychiatric Concepts in Nursing,* Philadelphia, J. P. Lipincott.

LANCASTER, J. (1980) *Community Mental Health Nursing: An Ecological Perspective,* London, C. V. Mosby.

LEONARD, P. (1975) 'Explanation and Education in Social Work', *British Journal of Social Work,* 5, pp. 325–34,

LOOMS, M. and HORSELY, J. (1974) *Interpersonal Change: A Behavioural Approach to Nursing Practice,* New York, McGraw Hill.

MARKS, I. M., HALLAM, R. S., CONNOLLY, J. and PHILPOTT, R. (1977) *Nursing in Behavioural Psychotherapy,* London, Royal College of Nursing.

MARRAM, C. D. (1973) *The Group Approach to Nursing Practice,* St Louis, C. V. Mosby.

MASLOW, A. H. (1970) *Motivation and Personality,* 2nd ed. New York, Harper and Row.

MERTON, R. K., READER, G. G. and KENDALL, P. (1957) *The Student Physician,* Cambridge, Mass., Harvard University Press.

MILES, A. (1987) *The Mentally Ill in Contemporary Society,* 2nd ed., Oxford, Basil Blackwell.

MITCHELL, R. (1974) 'Medical Model versus Social Model', *Nursing Times,* 70, 48, pp. 1851–3.

MUNRO, A. and McCULLOCH, J. W. (1969) *Psychiatry for Social Workers,* Oxford, Pergamon.

NATIONAL INSTITUTE FOR SOCIAL WORK (1982) *Social Workers: Their Role and Tasks* (Barclay Report), London, Bedford Square.

NEUMAN, B. (1980) 'The Betty Neuman Systems Model: A Total Person Approach to the Patient's Problems', in REIHL, J. P. and ROY, C. (Eds) *Conceptual Models for Nursing*, 2nd ed., London, Prentice Hall.

NEUMAN, B. (1982) *The Neuman Systems Model*, New York, Appleton, Century Croft.

OREM, D. E. (1980) *Nursing: Concepts of Practice*, 2nd ed., New York, McGraw Hill.

PARNELL, J. W. (1978) *Community Psychiatric Nursing: A Descriptive Study*, London, Queens Nursing Institute.

PAVALKO, R. (1971) *The Sociology of Occupation*, Itasca, Illinois, Peacock.

PAYKEL, G. and GRIFFITH, J. (1983) *Community Psychiatric Nursing for Neurotic Patients*, London, Royal College of Nursing.

PEARSON, A. and VAUGHN, B. (1984) *Nursing Models for Practice*, London, Heinemann.

PEPLEAU, H. E. (1952) *Interpersonal Relations in Nursing*, New York, G. P. Putman.

PEPLEAU, H. E. (1980) The Psychiatric Nurse — accountable? to whom? for what? *Perspectives in Psychiatric Care*, **18**, 128–34.

PERLMAN, H. H. (1957) *Social Casework: A Problem Solving Process*, Chicago, University Chicago Press.

PINCUS, A. and MINAHAN, A. (1975) *Social Work Practice: Model and Method*, Itasca, Illinois, Peacock.

POPE, B. (1986) *Social Skills Training for Psychiatric Nurses*, London, Harper and Row.

PUTNAM, M. (1981) 'Medical and Social Models', *Nursing Times*, 77, 19, p. 832.

RAMBO, B. J. (1984) *Adaptation Nursing*, London, W. B. Saunders.

RAPPAPORT, L. (1970) Crisis Intervention as a Mode of Brief Treatment, in ROBERTS, R. W. and NEE, R. H. (Eds) *Theories of Social Casework*, Chicago, Chicago University Press.

REES, S. (1978) *Social Work Face to Face*, London, Edward Arnold.

REID, W. (1978) *The Task Centred System*, New York, Columbia University Press.

REIHL, J. P. and ROY, C. (Eds) (1980) *Conceptual Models for Nursing*, 2nd ed., London, Prentice Hall

ROACH, F. and FARLEY, N. (1986) The Behavioural Management of Neurosis by the Psychiatric Nurse Therapist, in BROOKING, J. (Ed.) *Psychiatric Nursing Research*, Chichester, John Wiley.

ROBERTS, R. W. and NEE, R. H. (Eds) (1970) *Theories of Social Casework*, London, University of Chicago Press.

ROGERS, M. (1970) *An Introduction to the Theoretical Basis of Nursing*, Philadelphia, F. A. Davis.

ROPER, N., LOGAN, W. and TIERNEY, A. (1980) *The Elements of Nursing*, London, Churchill Livingstone.

ROPER, N., LOGAN, and TIERNEY, A. J. (1981) *Learning to Use the Process of Nursing*, Edinburgh, Churchill Livingstone.

ROY, C. (1975) 'A diagnostic classification system for nursing', *Nursing Outlook*, **23**, pp. 90–94.

ROY, C. and ROBERTS, S. L. (1981) *Theory Construction in Nursing: An Adaptation Model*, Englewood Cliffs, New Jersey, Prentice Hall.

RUBINGTON, E. and WEINBERG, M. (1977) *The Study of Social Problems*, New York, Oxford University Press.

RUSHTON, A. and BRISCOE, M. (1981) 'Social Work as an Aspect of Primary Health Care: The Social Worker's View', *British Journal of Social Work*, 11, pp. 61–76.

SHELDON, B. (1978) 'Theory and Practice in Social Work — A Re-examination of a Tenuous Relationship', *British Journal of Social Work*, **8**, 1, pp. 1–22.

SHELDON, B. (1982) *Behavioural Modification*, London, Tavistock.

SHELDON, B. (1983) 'The Use of Single Case Experimental Designs in the Evaluation of Social Work', *British Journal of Social Work*, 13, pp. 477–500.

SHEPPARD, M. (1982) *Perceptions of Child Abuse: A Critique of Individualism*, Norwich, U. E. A. Press.

SHEPPARD, M. (1984) 'Notes on the use of social explanation to social work', *Issues in Social Work Education*.

SHEPPARD, M. (1990) *Mental Health: The Role of the Approved Social Worker*, Sheffield, JUSSR, University of Sheffield Press.

SIEGLER, M. and OSMOND, H.(1966) 'Models of Madness', *British Journal of Psychiatry*, 112, pp. 1193–203.

SIMMONS, S. and BROOKER, C. (1986) *Community Psychiatric Nursing: A Social Perspective*, London, Heinemann.

SKIDMORE, D. and FRIEND, W. (1984) 'Should CPNs be in the Primary Health Care Team?', *Nursing Times Community Outlook*, 9 September, pp. 310–12.

SLADDEN,S. (1979) *Psychiatric Nursing in the Community*, London, Churchill Livingstone.

SMALE, G., TUSON, G., COOPER, M., WARDLE, M. and CROSBIE, D. (1988) *Community Social Work: A Paradigm for Change*, London, National Institute of Social Work.

SMITH, G. and HARRIS, R. (1972) 'Ideologies of Need and the Organisation of Social Work Departments', *British Journal of Social Work*, 2, pp. 27–45.

SPECHT, H. and VICKERY, A. (Eds) (1978) *Integrating Social Work Methods*, London, NISW.

STEVENS, B. (1979) *Nursing Theory: Analysis, Application, Evaluation*, Boston, Little Brown.

STEVENSON, O. (1971) 'Knowledge for Social Work', *British Journal of Social Work*, 1, 2, pp. 225–37.

STRAUSS, A., SCHATZMAN, l., EHRLICH, D., BUCHER, R. and SABSHIN, M. (1964) *Psychiatric Ideologies and Institutions*, New York, Free Press.

STUART, G. W. and SUNDEEN, S.J. (1983) *Principles and Practice of Psychiatric Nursing*, London, C. V. Mosby.

TRUAT, C. and CARKHOFF, R. (1967) *Towards Effective Counselling and Psychotherapy*, Chicago, Aldine.

TYRER, P. and STEINBERG, P. (1987) *Models for Mental Disorder*, Chichester, John Wiley.

WALTON, H. (1984) 'Medicine', in GOODLAD, S. (Ed.) *Education for the Professions*. Guildford, NFER–Nelson.

WARD, M. (1985) *The Nursing Process in Psychiatry*, London, Churchill Livingstone.

WHITTAKER, J. (1974) *Social Treatment*, Chicago, Aldine.

WHITTAKER, J. K. (1986) 'Integrating formal and informal care: a conceptual framework, *British Journal of Social Work*, Supplement, 39–62.

WHITTAKER, J. K. and GABARINO, J. (1985) *Social Support Networks*, New York, Aldine.

WOOF, K. (1987) *A Comparison of the Work of Community Psychiatric Nurses and Mental Health Social Workers in Salford*, Ph.D., University of Manchester.

WOOF, K., GOLDBERG, D. P. and FRYERS, T. (1988) 'The Practice of Community Psychiatric Nursing and Mental Health Social Work in Salford: Some Implications for Community Care', *British Journal of Psychiatry*, 152, pp. 783–92.

WOOF, K. and GOLDBERG, D. P. (1988) 'Further observations on the practice of community care in Salford: difference between community psychiatric nurses and mental health social workers', *British Journal of Psychiatry*, 153, pp. 30–37.

YELLOLY, M. (1980) *Social Work Theory and Psychoanalysis*, London, Van Nostrand Rinehold.

7
Social Work Knowledge, Social Actors, and De-Professionalization

Roger Sibeon

The purpose of this chapter is to identify issues arising from the use of social science as a knowledge base for professional social work. Following a brief introductory account of the relationship of social science to social work professionalization, a non-reductionist theoretical perspective is outlined as the basis for an empirical analysis in the main part of the chapter where it will will be shown cognitive-practico indeterminacy associated with welfare practitioners' use of social science knowledge has to be socially negotiated amongst diverse professional and non-professional social actors; arising from this, it will be demonstrated actors' perceptions of an 'excess' of cognitive indeterminacy is a significant factor in the movement towards the de-professionalization of modern social work.

Introduction: Social Science, Social Work and Professionalization

The relationship of social science theory to social work practice is described by Lee as a 'perennial' problematic in the historical development of social work's professionalizing aspirations (Lee, 1982, p.15). The term 'theory' is for convenience used here and later in a loose, inclusive sense to refer to formal social scientific knowledge whether this be formal knowledge of a theoretical or empirical kind. One of the first manifestations of social work's 'theory–practice' problematic was the attempt by the Charity Organizations Society (COS) in the late nineteenth century to define social work as the skilled 'professional' application of academic 'theory' to practice (Loch, 1906). Tensions surrounded this first systematic attempt to relate theory to social work practice, the COS leadership trying without much success (Bosanquet, 1900) to demonstrate that the sociology of the day, in particular

Spencer's (1877 and 1915) evolutionary Social Darwinism (Leonard, 1966, pp. 4–7), was a viable academic foundation upon which to build 'professional' welfare practices (Loch, 1906, p. xix). These and later developments, though there is not the space to examine them here, reveal that professional(izing) social work's search for an intellectual basis for practice created a 'theory–practice' problematic that in one form or another has persisted to the present day (Davies, 1981a; 1981b, p. 196; Lee, 1982; Satyamurti, 1983). In the post-war period, the search by professionalizing actors for an academic knowledge base centred upon psychodynamic and psychotherapeutic concepts (Mayer and Timms, 1969) rather than sociology, and at an organizational level some limited movement towards professionalizing objectives, occurred after the early 1950s (Seed, 1973, pp. 70–80). It was not until the 1970s, however, that these piecemeal steps towards professionalism came to fruition. The 1970s, particularly the early years of the decade, may aptly be described as the 'golden era' of social work professionalism in Britain (Richards, 1971; Editorial Comment, *SWT*, 1971). The goal of professionalism was brought much closer by the Seebohm Report (1968) which led in 1971 to the creation of the new 'professional' social services departments in local authorities. Other indicators of professional social work expansion in the 1970s included the formation of a national professional association, the British Association of Social Workers established in 1970; the movement towards a professionally unifying 'generic' mode of practice; and the unification of training in the form of a single nationally recognized professional qualification (the Certificate of Qualification in Social Work) regulated by the Central Council for Education and Training in Social Work following the creation of the training council by statutory instrument in 1971 (Seed, 1973, pp. 77–80). These developments during the 1970s led to the opening of many new departments of professional social work education in the universities and polytechnics (Davies, 1981a), prompting one commentator to observe '. . . the future of professional social work is its growing intellectualism' (Sainsbury, 1977, p. 213).

The large-scale entry of social work education into the higher education sector reactivated social work's 'perennial' theory–practice problematic, with consequences that in the next decade posed a serious threat for professional actors. The professional reversals that emerged in the 1980s are analyzed empirically later in the chapter with particular reference to the social construction and de-construction of professional cognitive indeterminacy. As a preliminary to that analysis its underlying theoretical assumptions are identifed below in terms that hinge upon possibilities for engaging in non-reductionist forms of social analysis.

Social Actors and Empirical Events:
A Non-reductionist Theoretical Perspective

In the sociology of professions, advocates of the 'trait' or 'core-attributes' model include Cogan (1953), Greenwood (1957), Goode (1957), Millerson (1964), Vollmer and Mills (1966) and Parsons (1968). An opposing, 'process' perspective is represented in, for example, the work of Hughes (1958), Bucher and Strauss (1960), Becker (1962), Freidson (1970), Elliot (1973) and Elger (1975). These writers identify a tendency amongst trait theorists to define 'profession' in terms of attributes (such as altruism, and a high level of 'tested' competence) highly favourable to professional actors, a tendency which results in a sociological depiction of professional ideology rather than reality (Freidson, 1970). Unquestionably, a taxonomic perspective in the sociology of professions has in practice frequently blurred 'trait' and 'functionalist' analyses (Daniels, 1975). However, these are two different modes of analysis, and provided they are not surreptitiously fused together a taxonomic approach need not involve uncritical sociological reproduction of professional ideologies. Indeed, in many existing critical sociological accounts alternative 'traits' are evident; these include 'professional privilege' (Portwood and Fielding, 1981), professional 'self-interest' (Perruci, 1976), exaggeration of task complexity through the creation of professional 'mystique' (North, 1972; p. 63), and occupational closure and monopolization (Berlant, 1975). If and where traits of this ilk can be shown to exist, the fact of their existence requires some explanation. A form of explanation prominent in the 1970s was structural Marxism. A notion that professional 'traits' are a dialectical, subtly mediated refraction of 'the interests of capitalism' is developed in Braverman (1974), Poulantzas (1975), Carchedi (1975), Navarro (1976), Ehrenreich and Ehrenreich (1979) and Esland (1980). In these analyses a recurring theme is that professions are '. . . agents of control for a powerful state' (Esland, 1980, p. 214). A more specific theme is that the teaching profession and health and social care professions reproduce capitalist labour in a 'docile' form (Sharp *et al.*, 1981) and perform social surveillance and control functions targeted against the working classes (Cockburn, 1977).

In ascribing structurally-given 'functions' to professions, reductionist theories of the type just referred to are seriously flawed and other, non-reductionist interpretations underpin the later empirical analysis. Theoretical issues relevant to the development of non-reductionist forms of explanatory analysis largely centre on finding ways of avoiding problems of reification. Harre (1981) in rejecting reified conceptions of social structure, lays particular emphasis upon the causal propensities of middle-range collectivities such as organizations or 'committees'. Organizations are 'structured collectivities' (Harre, 1981, p. 140), examples of which are government departments or other national or local public sector agencies or, say, voluntary organizations and professional associations; examples of 'committees' as a generic category include the Cabinet, or (as in local government) locally constituted committees of elected representatives. Middle-range collectivities are structured, 'relational' collectivities (Harre, 1981, p. 140) which exhibit 'real' relationships ('actual' interactions) amongst their members. They are also *supra-individuals*. In Harre's formulation, an entity is a supra-individual when it satisfies three criteria. First, it must be continuous in time; second, it must occupy a distinctive and continuous region of space or a distinctive and continuous path through space; and thirdly, it must have causal powers (Harre, 1981, p. 141). Non-relational, taxonomic collectivities (Harre, 1981, p. 140) such as 'society', 'the state', 'classes', 'men' or 'British passport holders' are not structured-collectivities (supra-individuals) with causal powers. To impute the existence of entities with causal powers *above* the level of the middle-range is in Harre's account a rhetorical personification of something which in an empirical sense cannot be proven to 'exist' (Harre, 1981, p.141). Hindess's rejection of personificationist conceptions of social structure is revealed in his definition of *actors*, who may be individual human actors or social actors such as organizations (Hindess, 1986a, p.115). An actor is '. . . a locus of decision and action, where the action is in some sense a consequence of the actor's decisions' (Hindess, 1986a, p.115). An implication of this definition when it is applied to social actors (or to Harre's 'supra-individuals') is that 'in so far as "societal" decisions can be identified, they are formulated by specific actors (governments and state agencies) or they are not formulated at all' (Hindess, 1986a, p. 116). Hindess rejects theoretical attempts to explain social action in terms of 'objective' interests presumed to arise from actors' structural location or membership of a taxonomic collectivity and where the (individual or social) actor is presumed to be subjectively unaware of having these imputed interests. As Hindess notes, interests are not structurally determined nor the 'fixed' or 'given' properties of actors, and interests '. . . that provide no actor with reasons for action can have no social consequences. They are effective in so far as they provide reasons for actors' decisions' (Hindess, 1986b, p. 118). A postulate that the concept 'interests' has no explanatory value unless it refers to formulated, self-defined interests pursued and acted upon by the social actor(s) concerned, may be compared with Leonard's (1983) Marxist perspective of social work. Leonard ascribes to social work certain 'functions' which reflect an underlying set of 'objective' structurally 'given' interests. According to Leonard, the proper role of critical analysis is '. . . *unmasking* . . . social work . . . and *revealing its underlying function*, the justification of the present structure of class, gender, and ethnic relations' (Leonard, 1983, p. xiii, italics added). In contrast, Hindess insists possibilities for engaging in analysis of empirical events are thoroughly obscured when the concept of social actor is '. . . extended to aggregates that have no identifiable means of formulating decisions, let alone acting on them . . . [such as] . . . classes, racial or gender categories' (Hindess, 1986a, p. 124).

The empirical account provided in the next part of the chapter will examine interactions between a number of competitive social (work) actors, including the Central Council for Education and Training in Social Work, the British Association of Social Workers, and the Association of Directors of Social Services. These social actors comprise, in Callon's (1986) terms, an 'actor network' (Law, 1986a, p. 15). It will be shown competitive professional and 'non-professional' social (work) actors within the actor-network engaged in intense struggles against each other in seeking to *define* and shape contemporary 'social work' in particular ways. To put the later account more fully into a theoretical context there are some specific theoretical issues that remain to be identified. Firstly, the empirical events described later were contingently produced within a particular (and relatively short) period of time, roughly between 1975 and 1986. This does not mean these events have no 'history', a point briefly noted at the beginning of the chapter. Where, however, any empirically demonstrated degree of historical continuity exists with regard to particular problems, ideas, practices, etc., this continuity is itself contingently produced and not the playing out of some historically or structurally determined 'necessities'. Hindess notes '. . . there are no essential structures . . . [any] . . . relatively pervasive or enduring social conditions . . . [are] . . . sustained not by some necessity inherent in . . . [the social totality] . . . but because they are situated in complex networks of intersecting practices and conditions' (Hindess, 1986a, p. 123). Secondly, non-reductionist forms of analysis explicitly reject the idea of a 'given' hierarchy-of-actors in which those at 'higher' levels always have a structurally 'given' determining or controlling influence upon others (Hindess, 1986a, p. 122). Callon and Latour in their empirical study of interactions between two competitive social actors (Electricity of France and Renault) are highly critical of the notion that social actors have an historically 'fixed' or structurally determined 'size' (Callon and Latour, 1981, p. 280). Actors contingently grow or reduce in size and power. Social actors, such as social work organizations or professional associations, expand by means of specific transactions ('translations') and according to the extent that they successfully enlist ('enrol') the greatest number of durable materials in the form of ideas and discourses, practices, techniques, laws and conventions (Callon and Latour, 1981, p. 284). Though the present chapter is primarily an exploration in the sociology of social work it is worth noting Callon and Latour's 'sociology of translation' (Callon, 1986, p. 196) is employed by Law (1986b) in an attempt to construct a 'new' and non-reductionist sociology of science; in examining interactions between social actors in the scientific community, one of Law's precepts is that sociological analysis '... should treat power as an *effect* of ... variegated and differentially successful strategies to enrol ... [other actors] ... rather than as *cause* of that success' (Law, 1986b, p. 5, original italics). Under certain conditions it is possible some expanding social actors will succeed in producing relatively long-lived asymmetries in size between themselves and other social actors, but where any lasting asymmetries of size and power occur this asymmetry is contingently produced and not the historical unfolding of a macro-structural 'script' (Callon and Latour, 1981, p. 286). Actor-contraction, a process identified later in the chapter as an outcome that faced professional social (work) actors in the 1980s, is also contingently produced through processes of interaction between social actors. Contraction may occur when the ascendancy gained by a previously expanding social actor is for whatever reason reversed. Callon and Latour (1981, p. 293) make the point that successful expansion is always potentially *'reversible'*; power defined as capacity to shape social events is a function of success in *irreversibly* enrolling and 'consigning' a large number of related ideas, techniques, and policies (Callon and Latour, 1981, p. 293) Thirdly, a particular instance of the empirical complexity and variability that surrounds social events is when actors' decisions and actions have consequences that were unintended by the actor(s) concerned. There are grounds for moving beyond Hindess's recent criticisms of the ways in which the concept 'unintended consequences' has been employed by some theorists. Though Hindess's specific criticisms (1986c) of the concept are bound up with his rejection of Elster's (1985) methodological individualism, Hindess's more general claim is that 'The tale of the unintended consequence is one of the more banal commonplaces of the academic social sciences ...'(Hindess, 1986c, p. 441). In a later text Hindess argues once the theoretical illegitimacy of macro-reductionism is acknowledged ' ... the idea that an aggregation of unintended consequences could explain anything about social structure ... [becomes] ... an absurdity' (Hindess, 1988, p. 25). In the same text Hindess goes on to say unintended consequences arising from actors' behaviour ' ... do not suffice to explain why they behaved as they did' (Hindess, 1988, p.106). Hindess's particular reasons for abrogating the concept are highly selective and do not lead him to consider possibilities for employing the concept in non-reductionist ways. In a useful theoretical account of the 'conditions of action' surrounding social actors Betts concludes ' . . . the idea of the unintended consequence is a *key* concept' (Betts, 1986, p. 44, italic added). Underpinning the empirical account in the next part of the chapter is a view that 'structure' as current social (work) context is partly the product of *the intended and also unintended outcomes of actions taken by previous, historical social actors and by the current actors at an earlier time*. Once these intended and also unintended outcomes have come into existence, currently ascending or powerful actors are (all else being equal!) better placed than others to 'retain', objectify and disseminate those outcomes judged by them to be in accordance with their perspectives and self-formulated 'interests' (Betts, 1986, pp. 62–3). Viewed this way, analytic use of the concept ('unintended outcomes') requires no recourse to teleological or reductionist forms of explanation. Included here is the notion that currently powerful social (work) actors are not only *selecting* from the range of existing opportunities in the situation that confronts them; powerful actors are also usually better placed than others, to exercise a *veto* (Betts, 1986, p. 57) to extinguish or 'damp down' other 'threatening' elements that may exist in the situation. This is not to say social actors are never genuinely 'creative' or entrepreneurial in constructing 'new' ideas or policies; nevertheless, in many situations ' . . . the more powerful actors are selecting innovations from the range that confront them, not creating them' (Betts, 1986, p. 63). Intended *and* unintended outcomes are, then, important factors in 'structure' as current context and important factors in the processes involved in the reproduction or change of the current context (Burns, 1986, p.14). Finally, these theoretical formulations incorporate elements of a performative ('translative') definition of social processes, though not to the extent proposed in, for example, Latour's (1986) critique of problems associated with the ostensive (or 'transmission') model of social structure and culture. Rejection of the reification inherent in structuralist theory does not require endorsement of an assumption that the 'conditions of action' surrounding social events are *wholly* 'processual' or in a state of total and endless flux and indeterminacy. Layder in a critical review of Elias's (1978) figurational sociology notes Elias constructs an ' . . . illicit dichotomy between complete stasis and complete flux' (Layder, 1986, p. 378) from which Elias selects the latter. This 'either-or' dichotomy is avoidable. Callon and Latour in their empirical work focus mainly upon the shifting, emergent, and empirically contingent nature of social events; but in arguing against the notion of a rigid, predictable social system Callon and Latour note that neither 'is . . . [there] . . . chaos' (Callon and Latour, 1981, p. 282). A relevant illustration of this point is the tendency, in the sociology of professions, for trait theorists to employ a static definition of profession. A static, unhistorical sociological concept of 'profession' ignores cultural and historical changes in the *meaning* of the concept (Freidson, 1983, p. 22). Professional(izing) social work actors are themselves 'readers' of these historical variations, though this, as noted earlier, does not mean there are *no* historical continuities in social work actors' usage and handling of the concept. Flexner (1915) titled his essay 'Is Social Work A Profession?'. A professional document issued many years later by the British Association of Social Workers contained a section titled 'Social Work — A Profession?' (BASW, 1977, p. 20). These two social work actors, separated in time and socio-political context by more than half a century, handled this question in ways that exhibit discontinuities but also some continuities of the kind referred to earlier as 'perennial' problematics surrounding 'theory–practice' and social work's long-standing quest for a professional mode of occupational structure. In the next part of the chapter contemporary constructions of these problematics are examined with reference to competitive social (work) actors' struggles to impose their own particular definitions of an 'acceptable' indetermination/technicality ratio in social work.

The Social Construction of an Indetermination/Technicality Ratio

The post-Seebohm expansion of professionalism was in part a product of professional leaders' success in portraying social work as an intellectually complex activity (Butrym, Stevenson and Harris, 1981, p. 8) characterized by cognitive indeterminacy (Butrym, 1972). However professional social work is permanently located in large-scale organizational contexts (Young, 1979, p. viii). Howe's hypothesis is that professional social work's 'psycho-therapeutic presumptions' (Howe, 1983, p. 77) have failed to provide an effective service to clients, as a consequence of which social work employers and administrators have 'taken over' professional social work in the search for increased efficiency in service-delivery (Howe, 1983, p. 77). Some writers, for example Wilensky (1964), note professional insulation from external administrative control is sustainable when, as in psychotherapeutic social work, both the cognitive inputs and the produced outcomes of professional activities are relatively intangible and shrouded by professional mystique. If 'everyone' (clients, politicians, bureaucrats, etc.) is able to judge-by-results, professional autonomy is diminished (Wilensky, 1964), a point recognized in Mackinlay's reference to professionals' efforts to '...remove certain activities from external observability and evaluation' (Mackinlay, 1973,

p. 77). Without *some* cognitive indeterminacy there is no 'profession'. However if the outcomes of professional services to clients are *wholly* intangible it is not possible to demonstrate professional effectiveness to other significant actors, some of whom may be powerful. Public sector organizations in varying degrees lay emphasis upon technicality, visible procedural knowledge and techniques, and externally 'assessable' criteria for judging the outcomes of professional interventions, in order to demonstrate organizational effectiveness and competence in the delivery of services to clients and service-users (Jamous and Peloille, 1970). As Collins observes, in organizational contexts ' . . . the strongest professions occur in the case of . . . [those] . . . which *are of the right degree of effectiveness and ambiguity'* (Collins, 1975, p. 342, italics added). Jamous and Peloille (1970) describe the counteractive imperatives of indeterminacy/technical rationality as a delicate *ratio*; if the ratio of cognitive indeterminacy to visible, technical instrumental rationality becomes too 'low' *or* too 'high' the professional-autonomy model is threatened.

Social construction and negotiation of the indetermination/technicality ratio in modern social work is illustrated in the following account of struggles over policy issues in the period 1975–86, the protagonists being social actors from three major social work 'constituencies'. These are, firstly, the professional(izing) constituency, where the major social actor is the British Association of Social Workers (BASW); secondly, the academic-professional constituency, represented by the Association of Teachers in Social Work Education (ATSWE); and thirdly, the employer's constituency, where the Association of Directors of Social Services (ADSS) is influential. The central actor in the actor-network is the Central Council for Education and Training in Social Work (CCETSW), this training council having responsibility for the national system of social work education and training. The contested policies centred upon CCETSW's proposals to 'reform' social work education. Jones (1979) and Bailey (1982) note social work education is a 'pivotal' institution which both influences and reflects wider developments throughout the profession; because of this, each of the major constituencies 'route' their perspectives and interests through social work training policies (Bailey, 1982, p. 12). The background to social work's policy struggles in the 1980s was a decision by the CCETSW in 1975 to introduce a new 'second-tier' qualification, the Certificate in Social Service (CSS) described in CCETSW Paper 9.1 (1975). The existing *professional* social work qualification, the Certificate of Qualification in Social Work (CQSW) remained as the 'first-tier' full professional qualification, the CSS being not for professional social workers but for '*social services*' employees in the local authority social services departments (e.g.

social work assistants, 'basic home services' officers (Billis *et al.*, 1980, p. 89), home help organizers and various other categories of social service workers). Following the creation of the social services departments (SSDs) in 1971 professional social workers were hierarchically ranked above social service workers in a vertical task-stratification model (Lee, 1982, p. 28). In 1975 the CSS ('social services work') was introduced as a 'new form of training' (CCETSW Paper 9.1, 1975, p. 5) that was less academic and more practical than the CQSW ('professional social work'). The CSS curriculum, and the criteria for teaching and assessing students' practical skills, were closely under the control of the employers who entered into a new partnership with colleges in the FE sector. The CQSW professional curriculum remained largely under the control of the academic-professional constituency in universities and polytechnics. The employers enthusiastically welcomed the CSS as a new, less theoretical training scheme more closely under their control and more relevant to practical skills training as defined by the employers. Actors in the professional(izing) constituency also welcomed the new practical training scheme. The BASW had pressed for the introduction of the CSS and in 1977 the BASW applauded CCETSW for creating a two-tier binary training system which recognized *the intellectual task complexity and therefore academic training required for professional social work ('CQSW work') was far greater than for social services work ('CSS work')*. The BASW for some time had been anxious to ensure the vertical task stratification model in the SSDs was reinforced and reflected in recruitment criteria as well as in the system of training and qualifications and the newly created CSS/CQSW dichotomy served *to reaffirm and symbolize BASW's arguments for a clearly demarcated hierarchical division between 'professional social workers' and 'social services workers'*. Later, it will be shown BASW's support for the new CSS/CQSW system had the paradoxical and professionally unintended outcome of creating 'new' conditions within the actor-network, conditions which severely weakened the professionalizing constituency while simultaneously strengthening the hand of other actors whose objective was the *de-professionalization* of modern social work.

After 1975 the employers found the new CSS practical training model so much to their liking that they exerted pressures upon the CCETSW to initiate a series of 'consultation' exercises (CCETSW Circular, 1982) with each of the major social work constituencies, these consultations later leading to three major policy reports issued by the CCETSW. These reports, in their shortened title form, were CCETSW Paper 20.1 (1983), CCETSW Paper 20.3 (1985), and CCETSW Paper 20.6 (1986). The reports proposed a major reform of social work education and training. The proposals were designed to ensure that, like social services workers, *professional social workers* would in future receive a less 'theoretical', more practical agency-based form of training. To achieve this objective it was proposed that, firstly, there should be far greater involvement of the employers in planning curricula and assessing the practical skills of social work students; and secondly, that steps be taken to abolish the post-1975 two-tier CSS/CQSW system in favour of a completely new 'unified' system of training *leading to the award of a new single qualification* (CCETSW Paper 20.6,1986). Responses to these proposals from social actors in each of the major constituencies led Sainsbury to observe social work by the mid-1980s had become riven by '. . . seemingly intractable conflicts . . .' (Sainbury, 1985, p. 9). The response of actors in both the professional and academic-professional constituencies was hostile. Pinker's (1984a) response to Paper 20.1 was highly critical. He protested '. . . the balloon has reached bursting point' (Pinker, 1984b, p. 18) and the publication of Paper 20.3 in 1985 and Paper 20.6 in 1986 led Pinker to argue the time had come '. . . to stop this initiative in its tracks' (Pinker, 1986, p. 21). Bailey stated *fusing together 'CQSW work' (professional social work) and 'CSS work' (social services work)* was untenable, and the CCETSW 'reforms' had failed to recognize the greater task complexity and therefore higher level of knowledge and intellectual training required for the former (Bailey, 1984, p. 59). Carter feared a loss of '. . . professional identity' (Carter, 1985, p. 28) and the ATSWE stated the idea of merging the CSS and CQSW into a single new, more 'practical' form of employer-led training rested on criteria that were 'incompatible' (ATSWE, 1984, p. 2). The BASW, which in 1977 had praised the CCETSW for having introduced the binary CSS/CQSW system, responded hostilely in 1984 to Paper 20.1; the BASW accused CCETSW of having '. . . the arrogance to . . . phase out CQSW/CSS on the basis of a back-of-the-envelope sketch' (Bamford, 1984). In marked contrast, social actors in the employers' constituency hailed the reforms as a victory. Harbert, a director of Social Services for a large local authority, described Paper 20.1 as '. . . *the most important document to be produced on the social services since Seebohm*' (Harbert, 1984, p. 21, italics added). Harbert rejected social workers' pursuit of '. . . status professionalism' (Harbert, 1985a, p. 14) based '. . . not on clients and their needs . . . but . . . on . . . the importance of professional power and prestige' (Harbert, 1985b, p. 15). The ADSS in welcoming CCETSW's proposed reforms commented '. . . in the past *academic* influence on CCETSW has been too pronounced' (ADSS, 1986, p. 2, italics added). Warner, the Director of Social Services for Kent County Council, wrote in 1986 that resistance to reform emanated from '. . . a shrinking cadre of professionals' (Warner, 1986, p. 15) who are attempting to '. . . insulate themselves from . . . the reality of 1980s style social services' (Warner, 1986, p. 15).

Warner described problems in persuading social workers to '. . . accept their accountability should be *defined* and their performance *monitored* and *appraised*. More appraisal and stricter accountability means *bringing things out into the open* — not something that professionals like . . . social workers like to do' (Warner, 1986, p. 15, italics added).

Employers' rejections of social work professionalism may be regarded as an indicator that the psychotherapeutically oriented professional casework model, a model successfully cultivated by 'expanding' professional actors in the 1970s, had by the mid-1980s become defined by powerful non-professional actors as a model that, in Jamous and Peloille's terms, had greatly 'exceeded' the indetermination/technicality 'ratio'. In 1987 the Government through the Department of Education and Science stated it would not fund the CCETSW reforms until further financial costings had been undertaken to see if '. . . the proposals are affordable' (Department of Education and Science, 1987). However many of the regional planning committees established in readiness to implement the proposals remained in existence after 1987 and there are signs of a *de facto* implementation of many of the assumptions contained in the CCETSW proposals. By the late 1980s the configuration of power and influence within social work and the social services had undergone a major shift; the optimism felt during the professionally expansionist post-Seebohm period had been replaced by a sense amongst social workers of belonging to a beleaguered profession marked by '. . . uncertainty and felt vulnerability . . . [and] . . . professional insecurity' (Small, 1987, p. 44).

In the non-reductionist theoretical terms outlined earlier, the outcomes just described were empirically emergent. The ascending social actors in the actor-network responded to and 'grasped' new opportunities that arose from the intended and unintended outcomes of the actions taken by different actors or by the same actor(s) at a previous time. Conversely, the emergent, empirically variable outcomes of the interactions had the negative effect for some actors of 'closing down' options that had previously seemed to be viable and attainable. There is only the space here to identify the main processes involved. Firstly, it was noted earlier the BASW actively supported CCETSW's introduction of the CSS qualification in 1975; this had the effect of creating the CSS/CQSW binary system which offered professional(izing) actors a new opportunity to reinforce a rigid distinction between social services work ('CSS work') and professional social work ('CQSW work') and in this way consolidate a vertical task-stratification model in the SSDs. However, secondly, this binary system had the professionally unforeseen consequence of creating other 'new' conditions and opportunities in the actor-network, conditions which enlarged the range of opportunities available to those actors who rejected the notion of 'professional' social work as defined by professional actors. These professionally unintended outcomes did not appear '. . . out of nowhere' (Hindess, 1986b, p. 120); they arose out of actions taken by other actors in an emergent set of conditions in the actor-network, these 'new' conditions having the effect of enlarging opportunities for some actors while simultaneously restricting opportunities for other actors. A significant factor following the introduction of the CSS scheme in 1975 was the employers' realization that their ability to 'control' the new scheme enabled them to ensure it equipped newly qualified workers with practical 'relevant' skills as defined by the employers and by senior agency administrators. When compared to the new practical training scenario emerging in the CSS schemes, the CQSW 'professional' curricula were increasingly perceived by employers as distanced, 'remote' theoretical programmes controlled by academics and professionals in the higher education sector. Once the CSS scheme had come into existence it became, so to speak, a new comparative reference-group for the employers. The emergence of an increasingly visible dichotomy between 'practical relevance' and 'professional intellectualism' was a crucial factor in employers' grasping a new opportunity to *redefine* 'the social work task' and then act on their newly formulated definition. Accordingly, employers began *appointing newly qualified CSS-holders ('social services workers') to posts that prior to 1975 had been the exclusive preserve of CQSW-holders ('professional social workers')*. Social actors in the academic and professional(izing) constituencies became concerned when they saw the introduction of the CSS was having this professionally damaging outcome (Carter, 1985, p. 27) and became even more concerned when it became clear the employers' movement towards organizational policies aimed at *blurring* the previously sharp dividing line between social services work/professional social work was inexorably propelling the CCETSW towards policies for a new form of 'unified' training that, in recognition of the *de facto* role-blurring taking place in the SSDs, would ultimately *abolish* the no longer sustainable CSS/CQSW training distinction. Professional power was further weakened by another emergent and also professionally unanticipated outcome that flowed from the introduction of the CSS in 1975. The CSS practical training model not only became a concept prized by the employers; it also had the effect of bringing into existence *a new pressure group* which joined forces with the employers in the struggle to 'remove' the power of professional actors. This new pressure group was the expanding corps of newly qualified CSS-holders, together with the newly appointed CSS trainers in the FE sector. The CSS holders argued the reality of the new division of labour in the SSDs, arising from their promotion to what had hitherto been professional social work ('CQSW') posts, meant a distinction between the two 'levels' of work was no longer relevant nor, therefore, was a two-tier CSS/CQSW training system relevant to the new organizational circumstances that were emerging in the SSDs. The CSS lobby mounted a vigorous campaign (Standing Conference CSS, 1985) for the same pay, titular status and career prospects previously reserved for professional social workers, and the lobby also exerted pressure (Standing Conference CSS, 1985) upon the CCETSW to act decisively and replace the binary system of training with a new, single qualification that recognized the reality of the changed organizational division of labour emerging in the SSDs (Parsloe, 1984, p. 113). The CCETSW influenced, though also had to be responsive to, this changing pattern of events and the role of the CCETSW shifted in the period after 1975. As the national council responsible for social work training the CCETSW defined its task as one of 'consultation' with the various parties prior to its formulating new training policies in response to pressures for more practical forms of training. The CCETSW initially attempted to secure some reconciliation of the conflicting perspectives that existed in each of the major social work constituencies (Bailey, 1982, p. 13) and in a rather convoluted, self-contradictory document published in 1977 (Wright, 1977) the CCETSW attempted to 'appeal' even-handedly to interests and perspectives held by all the major constituencies. Partly because its own perceptions of the personal social services were changing and partly through force of circumstance (in particular, the employers' reconstruction of the division of labour in the SSDs) the CCETSW's consensual approach to policy making became increasingly difficult to sustain as the configuration of power shifted within the actor-network after 1975. As power flowed towards 'non-professional' actors (i.e. the employers and senior administrators, the ADSS, and the newly formed CSS lobby groups) the CCETSW moved closer towards the interests and perspectives of these actors and by 1986, the year in which CCETSW's final policy report Paper 20.6 was published, leading members of the CCETSW were issuing statements that explicitly rejected professional actors' definitions of the concept 'profession' (Cooper, 1986, p. 18; Parsloe, 1984, p. 109).

It is not suggested the policy struggles described above have no larger context outside of social work's actor-network. In modern industrial societies, professional social work's psychotherapeutic 'mystique' is at odds with cultural imperatives that lean towards technical rationality, a cognitive mode identified in, for example, Habermas (1974), Arney and Bergen (1983), Figlio (1982), and Cooter (1982). The epistemological basis of social work's knowledge-mandate is 'normative', not 'scientific' (Halliday, 1985, p. 423), a factor which Halsey suggests weakens social work's claims to *professional* legitimacy (Halsey, 1984, p. 78). Gammack's defence of psychotherapeutic professional social work as an 'art' (Gammack, 1982, p. 20) dealing with intangible phenomena that like 'air and water cannot be cut or clutched . . .' (Gammack, 1982, p. 20) stands uneasily alongside '. . . *societal* pressures for concreteness . . . [which] . . . [exert pressure for] . . . an increasing focus on the *definable* element in . . . social work practice' (Gammack, 1982, p. 5, italics added). Psychotherapeutic casework is also a perspective not well received by clients who may have pressing material needs and require advice and services of a practical kind (Rees and Wallace, 1982, p. 155). Client perceptions of social work have a bearing upon the events described earlier. The interactions that took place in the 'actor-network' in the years after 1975 are in part a reflection of social work actors' differential readings of the 'causes' of the legitimation crisis of the modern welfare state (Offe, 1984). Reductionist interpretations of 'the crisis' postulate that the welfare state is threatened by the persuasiveness of New Right ideological rhetoric and that 'the electorate has been persuaded to give . . . support to a set of extremely damaging policies *which are not in their interests*' (Levitas, 1986, p. 18, italics added). This interpretation is not sustained by Taylor-Gooby's data (Taylor–Gooby, 1983; 1984; 1985, p. 20; 1986) nor by other data on voters' and service-users' perspectives; these data are available in, for example, Harrison and Gretton (1985, p. 47), Riddell (1983, pp. 138 and 239–40), Mishra (1986) and Butler and Kavannagh (1984, pp. 292–3). Mishra's analysis suggests service-users as 'voters' have rejected not *the principle* of state welfare (Mishra, 1986, p. 8), but rather, the particular institutional frameworks through which the principle is put into practice; in particular, Mishra identifies client and service-users' criticisms of '. . . professional dominance . . . [in] . . . the social services' (Mishra, 1986, p. 10). Against this background Harbert, the Director of Social Service, referred to earlier in the chapter, argues reform of 'status professionalism' (Harbert, 1985a, p. 14) is necessary if social services clients are to be discouraged from looking *outside* the local state sector for service provision (Harbert, 1986). Interpretations of this kind are rejected by some professional actors, an instance being Measures's rejoinder that Harbert's perspective pampers to 'consumerism' (Measures, 1986, p. 16). Measures's argument for an enhanced role for the BASW and for a return to the 'professional autonomy' model of the early 1970s (Measures, 1986) appears to be curiously out of touch with the current state of play in social work and the personal social services. A development that would have seemed unthinkable in the years immediately following the publication of the Seebohm Report is the recent movement to appoint professional managers, from industry, the civil service and elsewhere, to the role of Director of Social

Services (Francis, 1985; Whitehouse, 1985). The trend towards appointments of this kind, which provoke fierce professional objections from the BASW (Cypher, 1984), is on current indicators likely to gather further momentum (Francis, 1985, p. 15). Viewed against the context of a gradual erosion in the power of professional social work actors, particularly in the period since 1975, it is not surprising the BASW should have voiced its protest (Jones, 1986) when in 1986 the Central Council for Education and Training in Social Work announced it was appointing a new Director and also a new Chairperson — neither of whom were professional social workers (Maclachan, 1986).

Summary and Conclusion

The interactions between social work actors in the actor-network described earlier were empirically contingent and emergent, as also were the outcomes of those interactions. Though the network was not 'insulated' from historical and macro-social contexts, the actions and outcomes that occurred within the network were not 'necessary effects' of those larger contexts. It was shown social work materials (ideas, policies, practices, and organizational arrangements) were extensively redefined by 'non-professional' social work and social services actors in the period after 1975. The events that occurred within the actor-network centred upon the social construction and negotiation of, in Jamous and Peloille's terms, an indetermination/technicality ratio. Once the idea-influencing assumptions of Seebohm's psychotherapeutically-based casework professionalism had been 'breached', the word, as Callon and Latour put it, 'was out' (Callon and Latour, 1981, p. 290). In a complex interactive process involving actions, outcomes, and responses to outcomes, a new line of reasoning began to be unfolded. Social work actors in and around social work became enmeshed in interactions that reflected and in turn engendered a process of fundamental reinspection of assumptions that, by and large, had held centre stage in the social construction of professional social work in the 1970s. The outcomes of the intense struggles that developed between competitive social actors were not predetermined. As Hindess observes '... struggles over divergent objectives really are struggles, not the playing out of some preordained script' (Hindess, 1982, p. 506). In sociology of social work, a non-reductionist empirical perspective is critical of structuralist theories of social work, such as Philp's (1979), and is critical also of the reductionism inherent in epistemological idealism. Concerning the latter, it is not an argument of this chapter that social actors 'know everything' when they formulate their objectives and take decisions. Nor is it presumed actors' definitions and actions are always successfully imposed to 'become structure'. For one thing, the actor may not have access to the resources and strategies necessary for achieving objectives and the actor may in these respects be less powerful than other, competing actors. For another, the actor's intentional actions may have unintended outcomes which may later enlarge or restrict the range of opportunities open to the actor and to a variety of other actors. Certainly, though, actors do exercise choices and this is one of the reasons why outcomes are unpredictable. The diffusion through space and time of social work materials (ideas, practices, and policies) is empirically highly contingent by virtue of the material's 'passage' along chains of social actors with causal powers and any one of whom, as Latour notes, may choose to faithfully re-enact the material and transmit it to other actors in an unaltered form, or else choose to add to the material, or take something away from it, or modify and reshape it (Latour, 1986, pp. 267–8); and sometimes, in social work as elsewhere, actors may choose to (or have to) simply let the material 'drop' (Latour, 1986, p. 267). Whether particular actors in particular situations are *able* to exercise all of these choices is itself variable and, in sociology, something that has to be empirically assessed in a way that allows for the possibility of shifts in actors' differential capacities to exercise choice, a case in point being the interactions that developed in the actor-network described earlier. An actor's 'power' and capacities to choose and to act are not 'fixed-capacity' attributes determined by the actor's location in a social totality: these capacities are variable and sometimes the 'flow' from one social actor to another in an empirically complex, contingent and shifting configuration of events and outcomes. This is why nobody is able to predict with much certainty what might happen 'next' if contemporary professional social work actors renew their efforts to achieve professionalizing objectives that, though not always in the same form, have circulated within social work since the Charity Organizations Society first placed these objectives on social work's agenda.

References

ADSS (1986) (Association of Directors of Social Services) 'Editorial Comment', *Social Services Insight*, 22 February–1 March, p. 2.

ARNEY, W. R. and BERGEN, B. J. (1983) 'The anomaly, the chronic patient, and the play of medical power', *Sociology of Health and Illness*, 5, 1, pp. 1–24.

ATSWE (1984) (Association of Teachers in Social Work Education) 'Editorial Comment', *Issues in Social Work Education*, 4, 1, p. 2.

BAILEY, R. (1982) 'Theory and practice in social work — a kaleidoscope', in BAILEY, R. and LEE, P. (Eds) *Theory and Practice in Social Work*, Oxford, Blackwell.

BAILEY, R. (1984) 'A question of priorities', *Issues in Social Work Education*, **4**, 1, pp. 58–60.

BAMFORD, T. (1984) Chair of BASW, quoted in MURRAY, N. 'Two into one won't go or will it?', *Community Care*, 10 May, p. 21.

BASW (1977) (British Association of Social Workers) *The Social Work Task: BASW Working Party Report*, Birmingham, BASW Publications.

BECKER, H. (1962) 'The nature of a profession', in *Sixty-First Yearbook of the National Society for the Study of Education*, Part III, *Education for the Professions*, Chicago, University of Chicago Press.

BERLANT, J. L. (1975) *Professions and Monopoly: A Study of Medicine in the United States and Great Britain*, Berkeley, University of California Press.

BETTS, K. (1986) 'The conditions of action, power, and the problem of interests', *The Sociological Review*, **34**, 1, pp. 39–64.

BILLIS, D. *et al.* (1980) *Organising Social Services Departments: Further Studies by the Brunel Social Services Unit*, London, Heinemann.

BOSANQUET, H. (1900) 'Methods of Training' (COS Occasional Papers (Third Series No. 3) in SMITH, M. J. (1965) *Professional Education for Social Work in Britain: An Historical Account*, London, Allen and Unwin, p. 87.

BRAVERMAN, H. (1974) *Labour and Monopoly Capitalism: The Degradation of Work in the Twentieth Century*, New York, Monthly Review Press, pp. 85–123.

BUCHER, R. and STRAUSS, A. (1960) 'Professions in process', *American Journal of Sociology*, **66**, 2, pp. 325–34.

BURNS, T. R. (1986) 'Actors, transactions, and social structure', in HIMMELSTRAND, U. (Ed.) *The Social Reproduction of Organisation and Culture*, London, Sage Publications.

BUTLER, D. and KAVANNAGH, D. (1984) *The British General Election of 1983*, London and Basingstoke, Macmillan.

BUTRYM, Z. (1972) Paper given at conference, National Institute of Social work Training, cited in WILSON, D. (1973) 'The social work dilemma', *Social Work Today*, **3**, 22, 8 February, p. iv.

BUTRYM, Z., STEVENSON, O. and HARRIS, R. (1981) 'The roles and tasks of social workers', *Issues in Social Work Education*, **1**, 1, pp. 3–26

CALLON, M. (1986) 'Some elements of a sociology of translation: domestication of the scallops and the fishermen of St. Brieuc Bay', in LAW, J. (Ed.) *Power, Action, and Belief: A New Sociology of Knowledge?*, London, Routledge.

CALLON, M. and LATOUR, B. (1981) 'Unscrewing the big Leviathan: how actors macro-structure reality and how sociologists help them to do so', in KNORR–CETINA, K. and CICOUREL, A. V. (Eds) *Advances in Social Theory and Methodology: Towards an Integration of Micro- and Macro-Sociologies*, London, Routledge.

CARCHEDI, G. (1975) 'On the economic identification of the new middle class', *Economy and Society*, **4**, 1, pp. 13–23.

CARTER, D. (1985) 'Another blind leap into the dark', *Community Care*, 20 June, pp. 27–9.

CCETSW Paper 9.1 (1975) *The Certificate in Social Service: A New Form Of Training*, London, Central Council for Education and Training in Social Work.

CCETSW Circular (1982) Circular EDU/0055 18.1.82, London, Central Council for Education and Training in Social Work.

CCETSW Paper 20.1 (1983) *Review of Qualifying Training Policies: Report of the Council Working Group*, London, Central Council for Education and Training in Social Work.

CCETSW Paper 20.3 (1985) *Policies for Qualifying Training in Social Work: The Council's Proposals*, London, Central Council for Education and Training in Social Work.

CCETSW Paper 20.6 (1986) *Three Years and Different Routes: Council's Expectations and Intentions for Social Work Training*, London, Central Council for Education and Training in Social Work.

COCKBURN, C. (1977) *The Local State: Management of Cities and People*, London, Pluto.

COGAN, M. (1953) 'Towards a definition of profession', *Harvard Educational Review*, xxiii, pp. 33–50.

COLLINS, R. (1975) *Conflict Sociology: Towards An Explanatory Science*, New York, Academic Press.

COOPER, J. (1986) 'The making of a social worker', *Community Care*, 17 April, pp. 18–20.

COOTER, R. (1982) 'Anticontagianism and History's medical record', in WRIGHT, P. and TREACHER, A. (Eds) *The Problem of Medical Knowledge*, Edinburgh, Edinburgh University Press.

CYPHER, J. (1984) British Association of Social Workers, cited in 'News Item', *Community Care*, 6 December, p. 3.

DANIELS, A. K. (1975) 'Professionalism in formal organisations', in MACKINLAY, J. B. (Ed.) *Processing People: Cases in Organisatinal Behaviour*, London, Rinehart and Winston.

DAVIES, M. (1981a) 'Social work, the state, and the university', *British Journal of Social Work*, 11, 2, pp. 275–88.

DAVIES, M. (1981b) *The Essential Social Worker: A Guide to Positive Practice*, Aldershot, Gower.

DEPARTMENT OF EDUCATION AND SCIENCE (1987) DES letter 26 May to Chairperson, British Association of Social Workers.

EDITORIAL COMMENT, *SWT* (1971) *Social Work Today*, 2, 1, 8 April, p. 2.

EHRENREICH, B. and EHRENREICH, J. (1979) 'The professional-managerial class', in WALKER, P. (Ed.) *Between Labour and Capital*, Sussex, Harvester Press.

ELGER, A.J. (1975) 'Industrial organisations: a professional perspective', in MACKINLAY, J. B. (Ed.) *Processing People: Cases in Organisational Behaviour*, London, Rinehart and Winston.

ELIAS, N. (1978) *What is Sociology?*, London, Hutchinson.

ELLIOT, P. (1973) 'Professional ideology and social situation', *The Sociological Review*, 21, 3, pp. 211–28.

ELSTER, J. (1985) *Making Sense of Marx*, Cambridge, Cambridge University Press.

ESLAND, G. (1980) 'Professions and professionalism', in ESLAND, G. and SALAMAN, G. (Eds) *The Politics of Work and Occupations*, Milton Keynes, Open University Press.

FIGLIO, K. (1982) 'How does illness mediate social relations? Workmens' compensation and medico-legal practices 1890–1940', in WRIGHT, P. and TREACHER, A. (Eds) *The Problem of Medical Knowledge*, Edinburgh, Edinburgh University Press.

FLEXNER, A. (1915) 'Is social work a profession?', *Proceedings of the National Conference of Charities and Corrections*, London.

FRANCIS, W. (1985) 'Equipped to climb the ladder?', *Community Care*, 11 July, pp. 14–15.

FREIDSON, E. (1970) *Profession of Medicine: A Study in the Sociology of Dominance*, New York, Aldine Publishing.

FREIDSON, E. (1983) 'The theory of professions', in DINGWALL, R. and LEWIS, P. (Eds) *The Sociology of Profession*, London and Basingstoke, Macmillan.

GAMMACK, G. (1982) 'Social work as uncommon sense', *British Journal of Social Work*, 12, 1, pp. 3–21.

GOODE, W. (1957) 'Community within a community: the professions', *American Sociological Review*, xx, 1, pp. 194–200.

GREENWOOD, E. (1957) 'Attributes of a profession', *Social Work*, 2, 3, pp. 44–5.

HABERMAS, J. (1974) *Theory and Practice*, trans. J. Viertel, London, Heinemann.

HALLIDAY, T. C. (1985) 'Knowledge Mandates: collective influence by scientific, normative, and syncretic professions', *British Journal of Sociology*, xxxvi, 3, pp. 421–47

HALSEY, A. H. (1984) 'Professionalism, Social Work, and Paper 20.1', *Issues in Social Work Education*, 4, 2, pp. 77–84.

HARBERT, W. (1984) reported in MURRAY, N. 'Two into one won't go — or will it?', *Community Care*, 10 May, p. 21.

HARBERT, W. (1985a) 'Status professionalism', *Community Care*, 10 October, pp. 14–15.

HARBERT, W. (1985b) 'Crisis in social work', *Community Care*, 21 March, pp. 15–16.

HARBERT, W. (1986) cited in MEASURES, P. 'Professionalism', *Community Care*, 17 April, p. 16.

HARRE, R. (1981) 'Philosophical aspects of the micro-macro problem', in KNORR-CETINA, K. and CICOUREL, A. V. (Eds) *Advances in Social Theory and Methodology: Towards an Integration of Micro- and Macro-Sociologies*, London, Routledge.

HARRISON, A. and GRETTON, J. (1985) *Health Care UK 1985*, London, Chartered Institute of Public Finance and Accountancy.

HINDESS, B. (1982) 'Power, interests and the outcomes of struggles', *Sociology* 16, 4, pp. 498–511.

HINDESS, B. (1986a) 'Actors and social relations', in WARDELL, M. L. and TURNER, S. P. (Eds) *Sociological Theory in Transition*, London, Allen and Unwin.

HINDESS, B. (1986b) 'Interests in political analysis', in LAW, J. (Ed.) *Power, Action and Belief: A New Sociology of Knowledge?*, London, Routledge.

HINDESS, B. (1986c) Review, *The Sociological Review*, 34, 2, pp. 440–42.

HINDESS. B. (1988) *Choice, Rationality and Social Theory*, London, Unwin Hyman.

HOWE, D. (1983) 'The social work imagination in practice and education', *Issues in Social Work Education*, 3, 2, pp. 77–89.

HUGHES, E. (1958) *Men and Their Work*, Illinois, Glencoe.

JAMOUS, H. and PELOILLE, B. (1970) 'Changes in the French University-hospital System', in JACKSON, J. (Ed.) *Professions and Professionalisation*, Cambridge, Cambridge University Press.

JONES, C. (1979) 'Social Work Education 1900–1977', in PARRY, N., RUSTIN, M. and SATYAMURTI, C. (Eds) *Social Work, Welfare and the State*, London, Edward Arnold.

JONES, D. (1986) General Secretary, British Association of Social Workers, cited in Editorial, 'BASW re-states concern over new directors' qualifications', *Community Care*, 20 October, p. 5.

LATOUR, B. (1986) 'The powers of association', in LAW, J. (Ed.) *Power, Action and Belief: A New Sociology of Knowledge?*, London, Routledge.

LAW J. (1986a) 'Editor's Introduction', in LAW, J. (Ed.) *Power, Action and Belief: A New Sociology of Knowledge?*, London, Routledge.

LAW, J. (1986b) 'On power and its tactics: a view from the sociology of science', *The Sociological Review*, 34, 1, pp. 1–38.

LAYDER, D. (1986) 'Social reality as figuration: a critique of Elias's conception of sociological analysis', *Sociology*, 20, 3, pp. 367–86.

LEE, P. (1982) 'Some contemporary and perennial problems of relating theory to practice in social work', in BAILEY, R. and LEE, P. (Eds) *Theory and Practice in Social Work*, Oxford, Blackwell.

LEONARD, P. (1966) *Sociology in Social Work*, London, Routledge.

LEONARD, P. (1983) 'Editor's Introduction' in JONES, C. (Ed.) *State Social Work and the Working Class*, London and Basingstoke, Macmillan.

LEVITAS, R. (1986) *The Ideology of the New Right*, Oxford, Polity Press.

LOCH, C. S. (1906) *Introduction to the Annual Charities Register and Digest*, 15th ed., London, Longman.

MACKINLAY, J. B. (1973) 'On the professional regulation of change', in HALMOS, P. (Ed.) *Professionalisation and Social Change*, Sociological Review Monograph 20, Keele, University of Keele, pp. 61–84.

MACLACHAN, R. (1986) 'Changing the guard at CCETSW', *Community Care*, 9 October, pp. 15–17.

MAYER, J. E. and TIMMS, N. (1969) 'Clash in perspective between worker and client', *Social Casework*, **50**, pp. 32–9.

MEASURES, P. (1986) 'Professionalism', *Community Care*, 17 April, pp. 15–17.

MILLERSON, G. (1964) *The Qualifying Associations: A Study in Professionalisation*, London, Routledge.

MISHRA, R. (1986) 'The left and the welfare state: a critical analysis', *Critical Social Policy*, **15**, pp. 4–19.

NAVARRO, V. (1976) *Medicine Under Capitalism*, London, Croom Helm.

NORTH, M. (1972) *The Secular Priest: Psychotherapists in Contemporary Society*, London, Allen and Unwin.

OFFE, C. (1984) *Contradictions of the Welfare State*, ed. J. Keane, London, Hutchinson.

PARSLOE, P. (1984) 'The review of qualifying training: a comment', *Issues in Social Work Education*, **4**, 2, pp. 107–17.

PARSONS T. (1968) 'Professions', in SILLS, D. L. (Ed.) *International Encylopaedia of the Social Sciences*, London and New York, Macmillan and Free Press.

PERRUCI, R. (1976) 'In the service of man: radical movements in the professions', in GERSTL, J. and JACOBS, G. (Eds) *Professions for the People: The Politics of Skill*, Harvard University Press.

PHILP, M. (1979) 'Notes on the form of knowledge in social work', *The Sociological Review*, **27**, 1, pp. 83–111.

PINKER, R. (1984a) 'The threat to professional standards in social work education: a response to some recent proposals', *Issues in Social Work Education*, **4**, 1, pp. 5–15.

PINKER, R. (1984b) 'The balloon had reached bursting point', *Community Care*, 9 August, pp. 18–19.

PINKER, R. (1986) 'Time to stop CCETSW in its tracks', *Community Care*, 18 September, pp. 21–2.

PORTWOOD, D. and FIELDING, A. (1981) 'Privilege in the professions', *The Sociological Review*, **29**, 4, pp. 749–73.

POULANTZAS, N. (1975) *Classes in Contemporary Capitalism*, London, New Left Books.

REES, S. and WALLACE, A. (1982) *Verdicts on Social Work*, London, Edward Arnold.

RICHARDS, K. (1971) 'The new social services departments', *Social Work Today*, **2**, 1, 8 April, pp. 3–7.

RIDDELL, P. (1983) *The Thatcher Government*, London, Martin Robertson.

SAINSBURY, E. (1977) *The Personal Social Services*, London, Pitman.

SAINSBURY, E. (1985) 'Diversity in social work practice: an overview of the problem', *Issues in Social Work Education*, **5**, 1, pp. 3–12.

SATYAMURTI, C. (1983) 'Discomfort and defence in learning to be a helping professional', *Issues in Social Work Education*, **3**, 1, pp. 27–38.

SEEBOHM REPORT (1968) *Home Office Report of the Committee on Local Authority and Allied Personal Services*, Cmnd. 3703, London, HMSO.

SEED, P. (1973) *The Expansion of Social Work in Britain*, London, Routledge.

SHARP, R. *et al.* (1981) 'A case study of secondary schooling', *British Journal of Sociology of Education*, **2**, 3, pp. 275–91.

SMALL, N. (1987) 'Putting violence towards social workers into context', *Critical Social Policy*, **19**, pp. 40–51.

SPENCER, H. (1877 and 1915) *Principles of Sociology*, London, Williams and Worgate.

STANDING CONFERENCE CSS (1985) *A Revised Model for an Integrated System of Education and Training for the Personal Social Services*, Ballymena, Standing Conference Certificate in Social Service.

TAYLOR-GOOBY, P. (1983) 'Legitimation deficit, public opinion and the welfare state', *Sociology*, **17**, 2, pp. 165–84.

TAYLOR-GOOBY, P. (1984) 'The hitch-hiker's guide to support for the welfare state', *Sociology*, **18**, 1, pp. 88–94.

TAYLOR-GOOBY, P. (1985) *Public Opinion, Ideology and State Welfare*, London, Routledge.

TAYLOR-GOOBY, P.(1986) 'Privatization, power and the welfare state', *Sociology*, **20**, 2, pp. 228–46.

VOLLMER, H. and MILLS, D. (1966) *Professionalisation*, New York, Prentice-Hall.

WARNER, N. (1986) 'Social work: a cautionary tale', *Social Services Insight*, 1 March–8 March, pp. 13–15.

WHITEHOUSE, A. (1985) 'No professional has a monopoly of wisdom', *Community Care*, 22 August, pp. 14–16.

WILENSKY, H. (1964) 'The professionalisation of everyone', *American Journal of Sociology*, **70**, 2, pp. 137–58.

WRIGHT, R. (1977) *Expectations of the Teaching of Social Work on Courses Leading to the CQSW: Consultative Document No.3*, London, Central Council for Education and Training in Social Work.

YOUNG, P. (1979) 'Foreword', in CURNOCK, K. and HARDIKER, P., *Towards Practice Theory: Skills and Methods in Social Assessments*, London, Routledge.

8
The Case in Social Work:
Psychological Assessment and Social Regulation

David McCallum

In a larger work in progress on the history of social work in Australia, I am concerned to show how the particular methods of survey and investigation were productive of certain knowledges of the individual and the psychological make-up of individuals, which in turn became the object of a new person-centred approach to social work practice. In the early twentieth century, a different type of subject of social work was being formulated. A space was created in which statistical and survey techniques produced particular conceptions of the reality and 'truth' of psychological knowledge. Two prior issues are explored in this paper: first, the population question and the histories of this question, as well as the 'biologizing' of the individual apparent at this time; second, I want to look at an example of a blueprint and manual for social workers as practitioners of a 'technology of the social' (Henriques, 1984, p. 121) — Mary Richmond's *Social Diagnosis*, published in 1917 and reprinted seventeen times before 1955, and recognized in social work history in the United States as a major informing text for training in social casework (Gordon, 1988, p. 65). Casework emerged also as the key feature of a reformist social work practice in the post-war period in Australia.

Social work's own understanding of its past is largely affirming and celebratory of a reconstitution of social work practice within the new frameworks of scientific, psychological and psychiatric knowledges formulated during the first half of this century. In Australia, these knowledges are understood as producing a gradual transformation of the practices of a voluntary, untrained but well-meaning group of charity workers into those of a professional cadre of social workers, 'equipped with relevant knowledge about individuals and the community . . . [and] alive to the multiple causes of maladjustment' (Lawrence, 1965, pp. 30–32). Both in Australia and in Britain, the incorporation of these new knowledges was seen as tardy and unenthusiastic, leaving practitioners too long at the mercy of 'unadulterated intuition and commonsense' (Younghusband, 1964, p. 19). The Americans, on the other hand

> took hold of what the scientific study of living human beings had to tell them about the development of children, about the way people behave in relation to each other, particularly in families, about the characteristics of different kinds of people, for example, the ill, the delinquent, the solitary, the aggressive, the uprooted ... In short, they have used organizational method and applied scientific knowledge as the basis for developing the professional practice of social work (p. 19).

Yet it is not merely the characteristics of a technical expertise which are at stake here, and found wanting amongst the Australian and British social workers compared with their counterparts in the United States (Lawrence, 1965, p. ix). There is also the prioritizing of a new type of relationship with the object of social work practice, which required the closest investigation and scrutiny of the individual's character, the laying bare of the facts of an individual's life and relationships, the opening up of the individual to the gaze of psychological, medical and sociological inquiry. Again in the social work view of its past, these are the hallmarks of a new, progressive, interpersonal, humanist and even radical approach to understanding social life. This approach shared a similar framework and emerged at the same historical moment as the child-centred pedagogy in education, person-centred management of occupational selection and the individualized assessment and treatment of the delinquent and the inmate. In social work a new terminology was to take the place of such moral categories as deserving and undeserving, in the form of the case and casework, process, social diagnosis and what came to be called social network analysis.

It is not the intention in this paper to enter into debate on the question of the origins of a specifically professional approach to social work in Australia (Kennedy, 1988, p. 237). Such debates and the histories they produce need to be understood as histories of the present in which current social work practice is presented as legitimate, or else as merely an effect of class and gender relations. Instead, I want to begin to examine the formation of the individual subject of social work practice and the way in which psychological knowledges of the individual can be linked to new modes of regulation in the twentieth century. This type of analysis draws especially on the work of Henriques, Hollway and others, Nikolas Rose, and my own work on the history of psychological testing in Australia — specifically, that psychology has played a major part in the production of modern forms of individuality, and that the meanings and assumptions by which we understand ourselves must be understood as historically specific products (Henriques *et al.*, 1984; Rose, 1985; McCallum, 1985).

Like the extension of the medical gaze through the operation of the Dispensary in Great Britain in the early part of the twentieth century, as described by Armstrong (1983), the techniques of a new social work practice came to represent the Panopticon writ large, a whole community 'traversed throughout by hierarchy, surveillance, observation, writing' (M. Foucault, cited in Armstrong, 1983, p. 9). These techniques were another method of exercising power, requiring the social body to be monitored including both the normal and abnormal, and fixing a gaze on bodies that can be 'individualised by their relations'. So like the Dispensary these were techniques applied not so much on individual bodies as on the interstices of society, imposing on the spacial arrangement of bodies '. . . the social configuration of their relationships'. Armstrong's analysis thus becomes a description of the mechanisms of power which order and constitute the social realm itself; it is a mode of analysis

> for making visible to constant surveillance the interaction between people, normal and abnormal, and thereby transforming the physical space between bodies into a social space traversed by power. At the beginning of the twentieth century the 'social' was born as an autonomous realm (pp. 9–10).

Concern about the efficient and rational management of certain groups was part of what became known as the population question during the last quarter of the nineteenth century in Australia. In this period, psychological reasoning broke away from philosophy to adopt the scientific mode, to claim jurisdiction in the selection of immigrants, the organization of public schooling, and the assessment of delinquents, prisoners, the feebleminded and insane. In alliance with medicine and psychiatry, psychology sought to extend and refine the purely physical examination of the population through its investigation of the mind and mental operations, although it is important to stress that these knowledges did not speak with one voice and were often contradictory and specific to the location of their production. Relative to the weight of prevailing medical opinion, psychology asserted a progressive stand on questions concerning the abnormal and the management of a range of behaviours and conditions affecting the quality of the population and ultimately the survival of the race. In this sense, the formation of the individual in the first instance was made problematic not within the domain of speculative philosophy about 'man' or the individual in general, but in respect of a particular section of the population and in regard to quite practical and even mundane problems of administration and management (Minson, 1985, p.18).

Among others, Jeffrey Weeks (1985) in Britain and Carol Bacchi (1980) in Australia have drawn attention to an increasingly interventionist approach in the politics of the population question. The problem of the population was able to be framed in the earliest census data on births and marriages at the beginning of the nineteenth century, in the tendency of the poor to reckless overbreeding, thus producing their own poverty and becoming what was called 'swamped in vice and misery'. Against the Malthusian conception of immutable laws of population due to 'inevitable moral degeneracy', a new approach towards control of the population became evident later in the century in line with demands to maintain the imperial race and industrial supremacy — conditions which could not be met in the nineteenth century slum. Intervention emphasized public health, notification of births and more careful statistics gathering, correct childrearing and the removal of children from unsuitable parents. Good mothering became a national duty (Weeks, 1985, pp. 190–92; Abbott and Sapsford, Chapter 9 in this volume). In Australia, social efficiency and the defense of the Empire were linked to relatively progressive forms of population control and social programmes, reflecting the importance of a combination of eugenics and hereditarian theories, particularly as these were adopted in medical, educational and other professional circles (Bacchi, 1980; McCallum, 1984).

Histories of the rise of the population question and the so-called displacement of moralism by science have focused largely on the effects of Darwin's discovery of the theory of the 'survival of the fittest'. According to Richard Hofstadter, the theory of social selection adapted by Herbert Spencer during the last quarter of the nineteenth century was a representative translation of Darwin's ideas about natural selection on to people and human societies. For Spencer, the pressure of subsistence was '... the immediate and utmost cause of human progress'. The pressure of subsistence meant that a premium was placed on 'skill, intelligence, self-control and the power to adapt to technological innovation', which would sort out the best of each generation for survival (Hofstadter, 1945, p. 25). Another perspective implicates British imperialism in the extension of the 'survival of the fittest' idea on an international scale, such as that war as a natural law of history would proclaim the fittest of the 'races' (Semmel, 1960, p. 23). Again, in Gillis' history of youth, social Darwinism supposedly alerted an educated public to the danger of physical and moral degeneration, which justified an increased confinement of the young in schools and other asylums (Gillis, 1974, p.156), the latter ensuring that the worst of the degenerate would not procreate.

These histories have also tended to focus on the problem of legitimation of a social order, giving central place to the concept of ideology in the management of political consent. Russell Marks, for example, argues that in the event of the failure of the Protestant work ethic to be a plausible explanation for social differences in North America at the turn of the twentieth century, alternative means were sought to legitimate the grim realities of low skill, low paid industrial work. According to Marks, ideas about natural selection and an 'aristocracy of ability' served to persuade employees to consider themselves less bright and adapt to their fate in a genial fashion (Marks, 1980, pp. 86–122; see also Fitzpatrick, 1949, p.194).

Rather than focus on the conditions for the production of the knowledges and practices of social work as lying outside in some separate sphere like the state or the class system, I want to argue that we need to look for these conditions as arising from within the sphere of the production of scientific knowledges about particular types of individuals, in particular from medicine and psychology, and in the specific practices of population management. In the case of the child, the conditions arise from the convergence of mass schooling and biological discourses in the late nineteenth century. First, the gathering of children into classrooms as a product and the raw material of scientific inquiry in the form of a sizeable group of the population performing more-or-less regular and 'normalizing' tasks on an individual basis; second, the naturalization of the mind as an object of science permitting the calibration of the individual pupil, to be carried out by appeals to individualism as a natural state. In this example, according to Couze Venn,

> it is nature itself which becomes the origin and foundation; all explanations have to find their basis in natural processes. Additionally, they are the processes *as described by science*, so that the question of how we know that the natural processes are as we think them to be is answered by an appeal to scientific authority (Henriques *et al.*, 1984, pp. 144–5).

The purpose here is not to pronounce wrongness on psychology or to indicate its errors along the pathway to some final true knowledge of the individual. The point rather is to examine the insertion of psychology into everyday practices, the manner in which psychology produces individuals as objects of inquiry, and the effects of this production on institutional practices. This assumes that the effects of psychology are not governed simply by rules and propositions internal to scientific discovery, but rather that they are at work in definite applications of social management — the effects of psychology as a 'technology of the social'. The power/knowledge relationship is thus crucial to understanding the way psychology 'works'. The individual produced by psychology, and the individualizing techniques of institutional practices establish a system of mutual support and reinforcement.

So within this context and set of working assumptions, I now look briefly at Mary Richmond's *Social Diagnosis* book. I have described it as a manual for use in training social workers in the techniques of investigation, and Lawrence mentions it as signalling a turning point in relations between social workers and their clients: '. . . the clients' own ideas and feelings become the core of the diagnosis and treatment, and ''process'' became one of the most used words in the social workers' vocabulary' (Lawrence, 1965, p.11). *Social Diagnosis* outlines the role of what is called 'social evidence' in social work practice; that is, 'all the facts as to personal or family history which, taken together, indicate the nature of a given client's social difficulties and the means to their solution' (Richmond, 1917, p. 50). The book in effect is like a map showing where social workers would best go in order to obtain evidence on individuals and their relationships. There are chapters on the first interview with the client and then on other sources of evidence extending outward, so to speak, through family, relatives, medical sources, school sources, employers, documentary sources, neighbourhood sources, and social agencies including other social workers as sources. There follow chapters on specific cases where variation in the collection of evidence may apply: the immigrant family, desertion and widowhood, the neglected child, the unmarried mother, the blind, the homeless and inebriate, the insane and the feebleminded. The role of evidence in social work is made to correspond to evidence in legal terms, that is, its admissibility in constituting the individual as a case, and also in medical terms as constituting a case based on the accumulation of scientific facts. Its task is to provide 'the intimate understanding of character', as outlined by Octavia Hill as early as 1869 in an address to the London Social Science Association:

> By knowledge of character more is meant than whether a man is a drunkard or a woman is dishonest; it means knowledge of passions, hopes, and the history of people; whether the temptation will touch them, what is the little scheme they have made of their lives, or would make, if they had encouragement; what training long past phases of their lives may be afforded; how to move, touch, teach them . Our memories and our hopes are more truly factors of our lives than we often remember.

In the period of institutional transformation from a system of Charity Organization Societies in Great Britain, North America and Australia, mechanisms of surveillance and measurement of the population begin to appear, breaking down the anonymous mass of the population into individual cases and regrouping these cases around certain statistical norms. James Donald has described this 'hierarchic surveillance' and 'normalizing judgment' in relation to the effects of schooling on the organization of social relations and subjectivity around the turn of the century (Donald, 1985, p. 233). *Social Diagnosis* proposes an extension of the techniques already applied in the physical and mental examination of children in psychological clinics attached to the Children's Court in Chicago and from 1917 at the Judge Baker Guidance Centre in Boston (Gordon, 1988, p. 68), techniques which also became a regular operation in Australian courts in the 1920s (Berry, 1929, p. 24). The measuring, individualizing and medicalizing practices of the psychiatrists and psychologists produced in this case a particular 'reality' of delinquency, formulated in text books by the Chicago-based William Healy titled *The Individual Delinquent, Pathological Lying*, and *Honesty*, such that stealing was constructed as 'a symptom, not a disease, and that the physical, mental and social facts behind that symptom must be grasped and interpreted if we are to effect a cure'. This was to become the domain of 'the social'.

I want to conclude with the definition of the self announced by the psychologist James Baldwin, and cited in Richmond's book as the underlying philosophy of casework and social diagnosis. Baldwin writes:

> the thought of self arises directly out of certain given social relationships; indeed, it is the form which these actual relationships take on in the organization of a new personal experience. The ego of which he thinks at any time is not the isolated-and-in-his-body-alone situated abstraction which our theories of personality usually lead us to think. It is rather a sense of a network of relationships among you, we and the others, in which certain necessities of pungent feeling, active life, and concrete thought require that I throw the emphasis on one pole sometimes, calling it me; and on the other pole sometimes, calling it you or him' (Richmond, 1917).

The social was constructed in Richmond's book around the psychological theory of the 'wider self', located as a biological entity in the mind and produced through an organized system of connections, bonds and associations which was the sum total of the individual's life experiences. Richmond summarizes the theory in the phrase 'a man is the company he keeps'. This was to be the object of social work, the spacial arrangement of bodies, the multiple configurations making up the 'wider self'. According to psychologists like Baldwin and Edward Thorndike, their science would then be capable of predicting '... what any given situation or stimulus will connect with, or evoke, in the way of thought, feeling, word or deed'.

References

ARMSTRONG, D. (1983) *Political Anatomy of the Body. Medical knowledge in Britain in the twentieth century*, Cambridge University Press.

BACCHI, C. (1980) 'The Nature/Nurture Debate in Australia 1900–1914', *Historial Studies*, **19**, 75, October.

BERRY, R. J. A. (1929) *Report of the Edward Wilson Trust on Mental Deficiency in the State of Victoria with Suggestions for the Establishment of a Child Guidance Clinic*, Melbourne, The Argus.

DONALD, J. (1985) 'Beacons of the Future: schooling, subjection and subjectification', in BEECHEY, V. and DONALD, J. (Eds) *Subjectivity and Social Relations*, Milton Keynes, Open University Press.

FITZPATRICK, B. (1949) *The British Empire in Australia 1834–1949*, 2nd ed., Melbourne, Melbourne University Press.

GILLIS, J. R. (1974) *Youth and History. Tradition and Change in European Age Relations, 1770-Present*, New York, Academic Press.

GORDON, L. (1988) *Heroes of their Time. The politics and history of family violence. Boston 1880-1960*, New York, Viking.

HENRIQUES, J. *et al.* (Eds) (1984) *Changing the Subject. Psychology, social regulation and subjectivity*, London, Methuen.

HOFSTADTER, R. (1945) *Social Darwinism in American Thought 1860-1915*, Philadelphia, University of Pennsylvania Press.

KENNEDY, R. (1988) *Charity Warfare*, Melbourne, Hyland House.

LAWRENCE, R. J. (1965) *Professional Social Work in Australia*, Canberra, ANU Press.

McCALLUM, D. (1984) 'Theory of Social Differences in Early Twentieth Century Education in Victoria', *Discourse. The Australian Journal of Educational Studies*, **5**, 1, October.

McCALLUM, D. (1985) 'The Theory of Educational Inequality in Australia 1900–1950', Ph.D. Thesis, University of Melbourne.

MARKS, R. (1980) 'Legitimating Industrial Capitalism', in ARNOVE, R. F. (Ed.) *Philanthropy and Cultural Imperialism. The Foundations at Home and Abroad*, Bloomington, Indiana University Press.

MINSON, J. (1985) *Genealogy of Morals. Nietzsche, Foucault, Donzelot and the Eccentricity of Ethics*, New York, St Martins Press.

RICHMOND, M. (1917) *Social Diagnosis*, New York, Russell Sage.

ROSE, N. (1985) *The Psychological Complex. Psychology, Politics and Society in England 1869-1939*, London, Routledge and Kegan Paul.

SEMMEL, R. (1960) *Imperialism and Social Reform. English Social-Imperial Thought 1895-1914*, London, Allen and Unwin.

WEEKS, J. (1985) 'The population question in the early twentieth century', in BEECHEY, V. and DONALD, J. (Eds) *Subjectivity and Social Relations*, Milton Keynes, Open University Press.

YOUNGHUSBAND, E. (1964) *Social Work and Social Change*, London, Allen and Unwin.

9
Health Visiting: Policing the Family?

Pamela Abbott and Roger Sapsford

Introduction

It is now widely accepted that social workers are 'soft policemen' —
intervening in the family on behalf of the state — but it is less clear whether
health visitors also fulfil this role. Health visitors routinely visit all families
with children under the age of 5 as well as working with other groups. Their
major role is health education. Therefore, unlike social workers, they do not
intervene 'when things go wrong', nor are they responsible for assessing
eligibility for services or financial resources. Indeed, health visitors are
concerned that they should be non-judgmental and establish good
relationships with the families that they visit so that their advice will be
heeded. However, while this may be what health visitors think that they are
doing, they are nonetheless intervening in the family. In their mode of
intervention they can be seen as targeting the mother, working with
definitions of 'good' and 'bad' mothering and attempting to shape mothers
in particular directions. Their training generally leads them to work with a
particular view of what the family should be like, how mothers should
behave and the likely causes of poor health or lack of cognitive development
in children. In general they work with a set of ideas about the family and
child development which are patriarchal and middle-class. In this way health
visitors can be said to 'police the family'.

Health visitors work within a set of contradictions. They see themselves
as non-judgmental health educators. However, education is not neutral but
is based on a set of ideas — a discourse of what is 'true'. Indeed, the work of
the health visitor is yet more confused than this. In this paper we shall argue
that health visiting is informed by a number of competing and sometimes
even contradictory discourses. These competing ideas, which inform both
the self-identity and the practice, mean that the health visitors themselves,

those with whom they work and society in general are confused about what they are and what they do.

We shall attempt to demonstrate that the current situation can be understood more clearly if we examine the origins of health visiting and its subsequent development. It has its origins in the philanthropic visiting movements of the nineteenth century and the fears of contagion that developed as a result of the cholera epidemics. At that time its practice was informed by medical/sanitary discourses and was concerned with hygienic conditions of the poor. Subsequently health visitors came to be seen as key workers in training mothers to care for the physical well-being of their children (and their husbands). Initially their concern was with reducing infant mortality, and subsequently with improving the health of children. After the Second World War the role was broadened to health education work, but in practice they have continued to work predominantly with mothers and young children and have been influenced in their practice by psychoanalytic theories of child development. Pressure has been put on them to look out for both physical and mental cruelty. The theoretical training of health visitors includes some grounding in the medical, biological and social sciences. Often the different theoretical elements are contradictory and reinforce existing 'organic' (common-sense) ideas about the family, child development and the causes of ill health. The contradictions are reinforced by health visiting's individualistic mode of intervention and aim of educating the individual. Health visitors' problems of identity are emphasized by their medical/nursing background, the ambiguity of their role in relation to social workers, their domination by medical men and their aspirations to professional status. All these combine to produce a sense of need to justify their work at a time when the efficiency and value for money of professional interventions are under scrutiny.

Contradictions of Health Visiting

Health visiting was made a statutory service by the National Health Service Act 1946, the health visitor being referred to there as a 'family visitor'. It was envisaged that her duties would range more widely than just working with families with young children and that she would take on a range of health promotion duties. This is clearly expressed in the National Health Service (Qualification of Health Visitors) Act 1972. (These measures did not change the 1946 ones but became necessary when the health visiting service was transferred from Local Authorities to Health Authorities.) According to these Regulations the health visitor is:

> a person employed by the local health authority to visit people in
> their homes or elsewhere for the purpose of giving advice as to the
> care of young children, persons suffering from illness and
> expectant or nursing mothers and as to the measures necessary to
> prevent the spread of infection . . .

However, there has been considerable debate among both health visitors
and others as to what their role in welfare state provision should be. Dingwall
(1982) has suggested that the lack of clearly defined duties has meant that, as
new needs have arisen or been identified, it is health visitors who have been
called on to cover them. He suggests that their effectiveness, especially in
respect of work with parents and young children, has been limited because of
their non-directive style of work; that is, they have deliberately avoided a
'social policing' style of work, have had at best a loose management structure
and have had to seek client consent for their interventions. Furthermore,
health visitors have no legal powers and no command of financial resources.
They have a low social status and low rewards — they are one of the female
'semi-professions' described by Hearn (1982), dominated by one of the
established male professions (medicine) in terms both of the work they do
and the models within which they work (Rigler, 1982).

Health visitors are not unaware of the contradictions and problems of
their role position. In recent years these have led them on the one hand to
seek professional status and on the other to monitor and evaluate their own
work in more detail. They have been led to consider who they are, what work
they ought to be doing and the utility of their work as indiscriminate visitors
of all pre-school children. Part of this process has involved considering their
own professional qualification and their relationship to nursing and to social
work. Health visitors are all qualified (state registered) nurses with a
midwifery or obstetrics qualification who have taken a one-year health
visiting course, generally in a higher education institution with five 'O' levels
set as the academic entry requirement. (Some degrees in nursing enable
students to qualify as health visitors by the time they graduate.) Qualified
health visitors are now usually attached to a general practitioner — that is,
they work with all the families on a GP's list — and they may be located
either at the GP's surgery or on health authority premises. However, their
employer is the health authority, and they regard themselves as independent
practitioners; within the limits of their statutory duties and their
understanding of their role they have considerable discretion about when
and how they carry out their duties.

One of us (Abbott) has carried out research in the South West which
suggests that, even within the same health authority area, health visitors may

organize their work very differently from each other — although they all see their major responsibility as working with pre-school children and their families. However, how widely they define this role varies considerably. Some concentrate on health issues — the developmental monitoring of pre-school children and giving advice to mothers (rarely to fathers) on infant feeding problems, toilet training, etc. Others see their role as much broader and as concerned with giving advice on a range of social problems that may confront the families they visit, arguing that it is impossible to separate the social problems from the health ones. Others again are concerned to develop groups to provide social contact for young mothers, especially those they think to be isolated or not 'good mothers'. In the one such group that Abbott visited the health visitor had found a qualified nursery nurse to work with the mothers and had organized a series of speakers for the mothers — mainly on domestic subjects but also 'making the most of yourself' topics. Some of the health visitors undertook work with client groups other than pre-school children and their families, and indeed some of the health authorities were putting pressure on them to do so, especially with regard to visiting the elderly.

In Abbott's research there was a clear division of opinion among the health visitors about the possibility of undertaking this work and about its value. A few carried out a wide range of health promotion activities: visiting the elderly, bereavement and menopausal counselling and the running of anti-smoking clinics were among those mentioned. Others felt that they did not have the time to carry out additional work. Some argued that they could do little for the elderly as health visitors. Most felt that time was a major constraint on carrying out duties other than child welfare work. Some, however, felt that health visiting was and should be solely concerned with pre-school children and their families. One health visitor Abbott interviewed was giving up the job after ten years in post because she felt under pressure to change to a more social-work role. Another stated she was not prepared to take on a 'social policeman' role and would visit families only where there was a genuine health-visiting reason for doing so.[1] Conversely, others thought they should be involved in social as well as health issues.

However, one should not overrate the amount of autonomy that health visitors have. Meerabeau (1982) has pointed out that one of the ambiguities facing them is the stress on being independent practitioners in the training courses as against the reality of practice. Certainly all the health visitors in Abbott's research had a basic programme of visiting and clinic duties laid down by the health authority that employed them and were supervised by a senior nursing officer. The ability to take on additional health education work depended not so much on the decisions of the individual health visitor as on the area in which she worked. Those working in predominantly middle-class areas with GPs who limited the geographical area from which they were prepared to accept patients had more time to broaden their role than those practising in working-class inner city areas.

A further confusion concerns how health visitors see themselves in relation to nursing and social work. All health visitors have a nurse training, and many have worked as nurses before training as health visitors. Health visitors are generally seen as part of the community nursing team (comprising health visitors, district nurses and midwives), yet they are dealing with healthy people rather than with the sick. The majority of the health visitors whom Abbott interviewed did not see their nurse training as particularly useful in the health-visiting role. One said she still mourned the loss of her nursing skills after twenty years as a health visitor. Others did think their nurse training was essential and that they used nursing skills all the time in health visiting, although they often had difficulty in articulating just how they used the skills and knowledge. However, they all recognized that their job was very different from nursing.

They generally also made a clear distinction between their role and that of social workers. A key difference was that they visited all families with young children; social workers came in selectively, when things broke down or went wrong, to try to pick up the pieces. They suggested that social workers had training in case work which they themselves lacked. They clearly thought that there were health-visiting problems which they should deal with and social-work problems with which social workers should deal — although they also felt that these divisions were often blurred and that they frequently offered advice and assistance outside the health-visiting remit. Furthermore, as they visited families routinely, and as a consequence of increased awareness about and pressure to detect child abuse, they were on the look-out for neglect and abuse. One health visitor with whom Abbott went out spent some time talking to a four-year-old boy about how he had scalded his arm, while the mother was out of the room fetching a young baby. (Prior to the visit the health visitor had said she thought that the children in this family were to some extent neglected.) Some health visitors felt, however, that if too much emphasis was placed on surveillance, then this would reduce the effectiveness of the health visitor role, as it would make it difficult to establish a good relationship.

Another area of uncertainty for the health visitors is their status: their aspirations to professionalism, and their relations with the other professions and semi-professions with which they come into contact. The health visitors Abbott interviewed were all attached to a general practice (or several), and some saw themselves as part of a primary community health team. While some felt they had a good working relationship with the GPs, others felt they had a poor one. A majority felt that the GPs had no clear understanding of their role, did not refer appropriate cases and asked them to do jobs which they did not regard as part of their duties. A number, however, argued that the attachment system had considerable advantages over working a geographical patch. In the former situation a health visitor works with a small number of doctors, in the latter with a number so considerable as to make communication difficult or impossible. Indeed, the majority of the health visitors whom Abbott interviewed preferred attachment to the patch system and would have welcomed being part of a well organized and coordinated community team despite the feeling that GPs did not regard them as equal professionals but rather as subordinates. (See also Bellis, 1981.)

Relationships with social workers were also seen as problematic. While a few did feel they had a good working relationship, most did not. A major cause of concern was what they perceived as social workers' lack of respect for and knowledge of their training. However, the major problems seemed to be referrals. The health visitors felt that social workers did not take sufficiently seriously the referrals that health visitors made to them and that social workers wanted to wait until something went wrong rather than taking preventive action. Some felt this forced them into routine visiting of families that should have been carried out by the social services. A general complaint from the health visitors was that social workers rarely, if ever, contacted them to find out about a family; this was equally as true of families which were being visited by a health visitor as well as a social worker as of families that had been referred to social services and might already be being visited by a health visitor. Finally, health visitors felt that social workers did not appreciate how well qualified they were nor the nature of their responsibilities.

Abbott's research, then, suggests that there are three main issues facing health visitors: who they are, what they should be doing and what their status is. These are exacerbated by the lack of legal sanctions and financial resources controlled by health visitors and by their attempts to maintain a non-directive, sympathetic relationship with clients. All these issues have been discussed by social scientists in relation to social workers, who are more explicitly and readily seen as 'soft policemen' than health visitors are (see John Clarke, 1988, for a recent summary of this). What has clearly emerged from the debates surrounding social work is the ambiguity of social workers' situations. They are employed by the state, expected to carry out a surveillance and social control function, but also to establish a close, caring, supportive relationship with clients. It seems likely that in a climate of increased accountability and providing proof of value for money the ambiguity is going to pose problems for health visitors as well.

The Health Visitor Response

A glance through a number of issues of *The Health Visitor* and other nursing journals shows that health visitors are well aware of these issues and feel a need to discuss them. It is also evident, however, that there is no consensus among them. One of the main problems seems to be the lack of a body of knowledge peculiar to health visiting (see, e.g., Meerabeau, 1982; Robinson, 1980, 1985). Not only does health visiting lack a recognized body of distinctive knowledge, but there is also no clearly defined role to impart to the trainee. Health visitors deal with a range of problems that include health issues and welfare ones. Clearly this means that there is some degree of role ambiguity, which has been exacerbated by the attachment to GPs, but which arose from the change in their role from infant protection workers or well baby nurses to family visitors with the introduction of the National Health Service. (This is discussed more fully later in the chapter.) Hunt (1977) has argued that health visitors' lack of identity is due, in part, to their diffuse area of work; they are 'liable to invade the territories of other professionals . . . [who], in turn, have no basis for determining categorically which claims of health visitors are based on special knowledge and expertise and which lack foundation' (p. 23). The unclarity of their duties has left them open to being seen as central workers in a number of areas. Thus the Jameson Report (on health visiting) in 1956 argued that their role was to be health educators for people in all kinds of families and for the elderly, but with a special emphasis on monitoring child health and providing welfare support to mothers. MacQueen (1962) supported this view, suggesting that 'sheer numerical strength justifies the claim that the health visitor is both the main professional teacher of physical and mental health and the main medico-social worker' (p. 866). (See also June Clarke, 1970, 1972; Briscoe and Lindley, 1982.) A number of official reports have also suggested a key role for health visitors in specific areas. The Snowden Report on integrating the disabled argued that health visitors should play a central role in supporting disabled people in the community. The Warnock Committee on Special Education suggested that they should be the key workers for families with a handicapped child. DeAth (1982) suggests that the demands on the health visitor amount to saying that she should become the 'key community worker':

> The health visitor appears to have a pivotal role in the life of the community and of her clients which has been well recognised by all the caring professions as well as the numerous select committees. She stands at the interface between 'institutional' knowledge (with her understanding of hospitals and medical providers, health and hygiene, drugs and technology gained during SRN training and obstetrics training) and 'community' child-rearing patterns and expectations, life-styles and 'life chances', local folklore and the range or lack of neighbourhood services (p. 283).

However, there has been some reaction against broadening the role of health visitors and some recognition that it encroaches on that of social workers. The Report of the 1972 Committee on Nursing (the Briggs Committee) suggested that health visitors should spend about two-thirds of their time working in the family with mothers and young children and on other work related to maternal and child health. However, the wide range of work envisaged for them is also stressed in that Report. Health visitors

> will perform a range of functions in the areas of case-finding, support, counselling and health education. They will visit the new mother and baby as soon as the special skills of the midwife are no longer required and undertake supervision of all children both at home and at school, where they will be responsible for medical and hygiene inspections and screening tests and participate in inoculation programmes and teaching on health matters. They will have an important role in the provision of family planning advice. They will provide health and nursing support for the chronic sick and handicapped who are being cared for by nurses in the community. They will co-operate with workers in the personal social services department. They will provide health education in the home and elsewhere on all relevant topics. In these and other spheres of activity family health visitors will play an important part in the positive promotion of health.

Research indicates that health visitors do in fact spend most of their time working with families with very young children and that they see this as their main role (e.g. Clarke, 1982). Indeed, Clarke argues that health visitors should concentrate even more on young children and their families, but take on a wider range of tasks with this group of clients. The Court Report on Child Health (1976) also argued that the health visitor should concentrate on preventive health work with children.

However, the Cumberledge Report on Community Nursing (1986)[2] said that health visitors should be more selective in whom they visit and reduce the routine visits to homes of children less than 5 years old. Indeed, the Jameson Committee had warned in 1956 that 'one of the dangers facing health visiting is its very utility . . . if the field is too wide or the functions too diverse and demanding the future health visitor will be ineffective.' The 'universalism versus selectivity' debate also possibly conceals a social class element. (This is not clear in the Cumberledge Report, but the Report certainly suggests greater selectivity.) The health visitors Abbott interviewed thought that management was increasingly likely to put pressure on them to be more selective in visiting and were acutely aware of the need to justify their visiting of 'good' homes. One was extremely dissatisfied with her work because she said she worked in a middle-class area and the majority of mothers did not need a health visitor. Others made a point of stressing why middle-class families did need health visiting, usually arguing that the middle-class mother was over-anxious and needed reassurance. Some suggested that emotional deprivation could be a problem in middle-class homes. However, when asked how they organized their work it was clear that they visited working-class, 'inadequate' families more often than middle-class, 'good' ones. It seems clear that with greater pressure to justify their role, greater restraints on spending and new management structures the question of whom health visitors should visit will be voiced more loudly. Indeed, one health visitor reported that a recently appointed general manager had explicitly suggested that there was no need for health visitors to visit middle-class homes.

There remains, however, the problem of defining clearly just what a health visitor is. The Royal College of Nursing (1971; 1983) has been concerned to stress the key role of nurse training in preparation for health visiting. However, it was not in fact until 1962 that nurse training was made a prerequisite for entry to training as a health visitor and health visiting became clearly identified as a part of nursing — an identity more clearly established by the incorporation of the Council for the Education and Training of Health Visitors into the Nursing and Midwifery Council in 1980. Health visitors themselves have been less ready to identify themselves as nurses. In 1970 the Health Visitors' Association argued that health visiting was an independent profession, linked to nursing and social work but separate and essentially different from either. However, changes in both the control of health visitor training and the health service administration have made the identification of health visiting as part of nursing more certain. The implementation in 1974 of the National Health Service Reorganisation Act 1973 resulted in the unification of hospital and community nursing; health visitors escaped their domination by medical officers but were now likely to be dominated by hospital-oriented managers — a process exacerbated by changes in the 1980s.

Nurse training, with its curative orientation, often makes it difficult for health visitors to adjust to a role as health educators and preventive health workers. It also has implications for their relationship with doctors. When local authorities first began to employ health visitors, the latter worked under the direction of medical officers of health, and this continued until 1974. As a result, according to Robinson (1985), they shared the MOHs' low status. Certainly health visitors were not highly regarded by general practitioners in the period after World War II, and in some areas this led to the advocation of 'attachment'. It was thought that this would enable GPs to understand and appreciate better the important work undertaken by the health visitors (Jefferys, 1965). However, the identification of health visitors with nurses, the associated low status and the assumption of authority by doctors have meant that there continues to be an uneasy relationship between doctors and health visitors. Doctors are uncertain as to the exact role of health visitors and probably in some cases suspicious that the health visitor is attempting to usurp the GP's authority in the advice given to families (see Cartlidge, 1985; Draper *et al.*, 1984).

The final area of role confusion for health visitors is the relationship of their work to that of social workers. This is not just a problem of the relationship between the two groups, but one of a lack of clarity about the relationship of the 'disciplines'. Official reports since 1946 have failed to clarify this relationship. The problems are exacerbated by a lack of understanding by social workers of the health visitors' training and a feeling among the latter that social workers devalue their qualifications and see them as inferior. As Robinson (1985) points out, the establishment in 1948 by local authorities of children's committees and the employment of children's officers was an aspect of this. The recommendation that children's officers should be social science graduates with experience of child work highlighted the low status of health visitors at the time, with a non-graduate background and a training that still perpetuated the medical morality of the 1920s. While not all social workers have graduate qualifications (and some employed social workers are 'unqualified'), they have adopted a professional identity that places them as superior to health visitors. This is exacerbated by what health visitors see as social workers' ability to select the cases with which they will deal and refuse to accept the concerns of health visitors as necessarily valid.

In recent years, along with nurses, health visitors have sought to increase their professional standing and to argue that there is a distinct knowledge base for health visiting and that this can be used in a systematic manner — the Health Visiting Process.[3] However, a major problem here is the lack of a theory of health visiting (Robinson, 1980). Health visitors' education includes knowledge from a number of disciplines, including medicine, biology and the social sciences. The different theoretical perspectives taught may actually contradict each other, leading to a high degree of pragmatism (see, e.g., Dingwall, 1979). Also, there is no one model of health visiting practice, as this depends on how the theoretical knowledge is translated into actions by the health visitors. Robinson argues that there are two possible models of practice: a clinical model oriented to health problems, and a relationship-centred approach. The closer alignment of health visiting with nursing means that moves to increase professional standing by advanced training must be seen within the context of changes in nurse education generally. Here there are moves to increase the number of nursing graduates both from first degrees in nursing and from post-registration nursing degrees, and for schools of nursing to work in close contact with local institutions of higher education. Suggestions for nurse training in *Nursing 2000* (1985)[4] and the Cumberledge Report (1986) can also be seen as pushing for enhanced levels of qualification. However, at the same time the question is being raised of whether professional status is really what should be being aimed for (e.g. Salvage, 1985; Schrock, 1982; Oakley, 1984). More importantly, other factors are pushing health visitors in the opposite direction. Moves towards greater accountability and new management structures indicate that the work of health visitors may be more closely monitored in the future. Furthermore, in many areas they will no longer be managed by qualified health visitors. The introduction of structured visiting and more detailed and structured record-keeping may actually de-skill health visiting, taking away from the health visitor the right to use her own judgment on frequency and timing of visits.

Social Policing

We have stressed that while health visitors are uncertain about their role, a number of key ideas have informed their practice. Paramount among these have been the deliberate avoidance of a 'social policing' style of work, working with client consent and a loose management structure giving them apparent freedom in arranging their own work. Underlying these is the fact that the health visitor has no legal powers and commands no resources. However, it is important to remember that health visitors play a role on behalf of the state in monitoring and preventing breakdown. They have a key surveillance role in ensuring 'normal' child development, encouraging certain patterns of mothering and child care and identifying 'poor', 'bad', 'inadequate' mothers. In this way they may have an important function in the system of social control. Two aspects of this have been discussed in the health visiting literature. One concerns the individualistic approach of health visitors to health problems, and the other the middle-class, patriarchal assumptions that underlie their practice.

Rigler (1982) has argued that, because of their nursing background and because they work with general practitioners, health visitors have an inbuilt bias towards personalizing health and welfare problems. This bias is increased by the fact that health visiting is a personalized interaction, dealing with individual mothers. This means that health visitors tend to ignore the social causes of personal troubles. We suggest that this tendency to work with an individualistic perspective is compounded by child development knowledge which health visitors learn on their specialized training courses and the stress that midwives and health visitors place on mother–child bonding and 'normal' mother–child interaction. Furthermore, psychological theories of child development tend to assume the 'normal' family, even if this is not made explicit. Thus the family, and by implication the mother, is seen as a key agent of socialization of children and as the provider of the stability and nurturance necessary for healthy mental development. This individualizing tendency is increased by the continuing dominance of psychological theories of child abuse (see Parton, 1985, for a critical review of this literature). It seems that while health visitors may be introduced to the wider literature on the social, economic and political causes of ill health and social problems, the personalized nature of their interaction, their nurse training and the child development literature have more impact on their practice. Their mode of interaction is to teach mothers (families) to care for their children and other family members in more appropriate ways.

Jean Orr (1986) has taken up the issue of health visiting practice and mode of interaction from a feminist perspective. She argues that health-visitor training reinforces middle-class, patriarchal attitudes to the family already held by the trainees — that is, they are taught that the ideal-typical nuclear family is biologically given and socially necessary as the context for normal child development. She argues that rather than helping women to care for their own and their children's health, the health visitor's interactions are designed to reinforce/maintain/create the patriarchal nuclear family. This includes expecting particular patterns of child development (based on middle-class values and expectations), with the implication that if the child cannot pass the test then it is the mother's fault, and reinforcing the view that mothers are responsible for the health, nurturance and cognitive development of their children. Families that do not conform to the norm of the ideal-typical nuclear family are seen as deviant and as needing more frequent health-visitor input and more advice on child care and child development.

However, Orr is raising an issue that goes beyond the health visitor's role in helping to maintain the subordinate position of women. She is pointing to the contradiction in the title 'family visitor'. While health visitors are supposed to provide health education for a variety of families, in fact they prioritize the interests of children, in terms both of the allocation of their time and of the way in which they intervene in families. As Denise Riley (1983) has pointed out, social policy aimed at the family actually addresses individual members — men, women, children — separately. Women have been targeted as the carers for children on behalf of the nation; the interests of children have been prioritized over those of mothers (see also Abbott and Sapsford, 1987). This is seen clearly both in the publicity campaigns after the Boer War, when mothers were admonished for not caring adequately for their children — while less attention was paid to their own health and well-being — and after the Second World War, when women were encouraged to have more children and to give up paid work outside the home because their 'real' work as mothers took priority. Children's needs (and those of men) took precedence over those of mothers. Health visitors continue to work with a stock of knowledge that demands a particular role of the mother — that of caring full time for her children. The health needs of mothers, when they conflict with those of their children, are seen as less important, if they are considered at all. In a sense Orr is arguing that health visitors do not consider the needs of mothers at all — they see them just as mothers and focus their concern on the children.

However, one should be careful not to be critical of interventions in the family without taking into account issues of power. Obviously in some senses the professional intervening in the family possesses the power, but this power is used to an extent on behalf of the less powerful. By taking the position of women, as Orr does, it is possible to ignore the position of children, and by definition children are the least powerful members of families. Health visitors intervene in the family at least in part to protect children. As Wise (1985) has argued with respect to social workers, it is essential that they do act as agents of social control and in so doing protect the most vulnerable members of society — children. This does not mean that health visitors cannot work with mothers and take a feminist stance in challenging the hegemonic role that doctors claim over them and their work. However, it is necessary for them to think through the way this challenges their organic ideas about the family and the role of women in society.

Health visitors, then, work within a familial ideology and an individualistic model of the causation of health and social problems. Specifically, given that they work predominantly with families with young children, they reinforce and try to establish particular patterns of child care and family formation. In undertaking this role they work predominantly with mothers and tend also to reinforce culturally dominant views of the role of wives and mothers. Given that health visitors have some contact with the vast majority of families with pre-school children, they must play an important part in maintaining existing forms of mothering and child care and consequently in the social control of women (see also David, 1985). The importance of this aspect of health visiting — albeit that it may well be a 'hidden agenda' of which health visitors themselves are not aware, family ideology being part of their taken-for-granted stock of knowledge — is clearly demonstrated when we look at the history of health visiting. Indeed, an examination of the history of the health visiting services goes a long way towards enabling us to understand the ambiguities and problems that confront health visitors in the 1980s.

Foucault and the Power of Knowledge

In our reading of the history of health visiting we are heavily influenced by the ideas of Michel Foucault, especially those developed in his later work (e.g. Foucault, 1975; 1976; see also Smart, 1985; Rose, 1985; Hewitt, 1983).[5] In his later work Foucault was concerned to explore the ways in which modern Western society has become increasingly disciplined, regulated and kept under surveillance. The welfare state and its agents (doctors, nurses, health visitors, social workers, etc.) play an important role in this process.

Foucault has analyzed the relationship between certain medical and social science discourses and the exercise of power in modern Western societies. He is concerned to examine the relationship between discourses, practice and professional groups. He suggests that power/knowledge has become organized around enquiries into the body (of the individual) and bodies (of the population). The body has become both the object and the target of power. Biopolitics is his term for the development of concern about the health of individuals and populations and the power strategies used to normalize individuals and populations in this respect. Scientific/medical discourses and the associated exercise of professional power were involved in the growth of surveillance of societies through the exercise of discipline over the body and the population. From the eighteenth century onwards medical men, philanthropists, social workers, health visitors, etc., become the new receivers of confession — the collectors of the inner thoughts, attitudes and assumptions of private citizens. The bureaucratic questionnaire became the linkage between the individual citizen and the public world of politics and administration. The regulating state regulates the individual citizen. As mind is assimilated to body with the development of a discourse of psychological regulation in the twentieth century (Rose, 1985; 1989) the emphasis has shifted from physical and moral health to mental health, and surveillance has become correspondingly more detailed and intrusive (Sapsford, 1990).

Power for Foucault resides in the claim to truth, and what is understood by 'truth' in medicine and the social sciences has played a large part as justification for the exercise of social control. Medicine and the social sciences, including their psychological/psychoanalytic branches, claim the arbitration of truth because of their scientific nature (as branches of the overall 'discourse of positivism' which has won the battle for truth in the modern world), and to the extent that these new discourses became established as 'having truth' they acquired power. Thus the advances in social medicine, the social sciences, biology and psychiatry provided a power/knowledge base for a large group of professions which intervened in the lives of individuals and populations. This led to, and its growth was stimulated by, new methods of surveying the population and the routine collection of statistical information about population growth — making it possible to monitor the birth rate. Thus the population was created as an object of government and as a subject of needs, through the creation of the means to measure and monitor it. The concern with the health of the population arose out of new discourses and gave rise to a range of new tactics and techniques of power, concerned with the health and well-being of individuals and of the population as a whole. The tactics of intervention are seldom direct and coercive; more often they involve teaching people (e.g. mothers) how to achieve goals which they and the experts 'agree' are desirable. In accepting the goals and the advice, however, mothers accept the expert's definition of the situation, and so the expert comes to determine the nature of the mother's social world. 'Pastoral' power — the power entailed in advising, counselling and facilitating — is no less effective than coercive power in determining how people shall understand and live in the social world.

The Development of Health Visiting

Health visitors were one group of the agents of pastoral power that became established in late nineteenth- and early twentieth-century Britain. The origins of health visiting and the conditions for the existence of health visitors can be located in biopolitics and the medical and hygiene discourse that developed in nineteenth-century England. Health visitors played an important role in normalizing the working-class family, and especially the mother, in the early twentieth century (see Davin, 1978; Rowan, 1985). The basis of their power at that time was the medical discourse on infant care, diet and hygiene. Subsequently health visitors have extended their knowledge base to include material on the psychological and biological growth of the normal child. While the focus of attention was the infant and child, the major target of normalization was the working-class mother. Health visitors used their power/knowledge to create a certain type of mother — the modern mother whose major focus of concern is the health and well-being of her family and specifically her child(ren). With the increased influence of psychology/psychiatry and the consequent growth in the complexity of the mother's task, what was in origin a form of control of working-class mothers has become applied to all mothers, and a movement that in origin tried to impose middle-class norms on working-class mothers has now come to exercise control over middle-class mothers as well (Sapsford, 1990).

Health visiting has its historical roots in the nineteenth-century visiting movements (Prockoska, 1980), with their concern about the condition of the poor and the regulation of the population (Bland and Mort, 1984). Part of this concern was with the conditions in which the poor lived, which were seen as a potential source of contagious diseases as well as of social and moral corruption. These movements were influenced by a number of different motivations and interests, however. Evangelicalism, with its emphasis on personal salvation and the need to save the immoral and prevent immorality was one clear influence. Banks (1981) has argued that the involvement of middle-class women was an outcome of growing feminism in Victorian England; philanthropic good works were an outlet for upper middle-class women who were no longer satisfied with their roles as wives and mothers but who continued to share Victorian values as to the appropriate roles for women. These Visiting Societies were often made up of male committees using (unpaid) female visitors, although some were set up and run by women. Often the major motivation for visiting the poor was religion, but the visitors frequently undertook nursing duties and gave advice on hygiene, child-care, cooking, etc. These societies were philanthropic; that is, they were concerned with personal conduct and morality. They aimed to correct and reform the poor by the giving of advice. Their philosophy was based on ideas of self-reliance and self-help rather than of charity (see Donzelot, 1977, for an extended discussion).

At the same time there was a growing concern about the health of the poor and a realization that a healthy workforce was a more efficient one (see, e.g., Chadwick, 1842). Specific concern was focused on hygiene, urged on by the cholera epidemics and the fears of the middle class that contagion would spread from the working-class areas of the towns (Wohl, 1986). A medical discourse centring on cleanliness developed, arguing not only for social reform but also for the working class to be instructed in matters of cleanliness (see Dowling, 1963; Wohl, 1986). Medical men played an important role both in advocating public health reforms and in the Health of Towns Association, established in 1884. In Newcastle, one founding member of a Sanitary Association, a medical man, argued that the chief object was

> to diffuse among the inhabitants of the district the valuable information elicited by recent enquiries, and the advancement of science as to the physical and moral evils that result from the present defective sanitary conditions of these towns and to impress on the working class, in particular, by every available means, a conviction of the injurious influences exercised upon their health and moral condition by inattention to . . . the cleanliness of their persons and homes (Robinson, 1849, p. 8).

The discourses surrounding hygiene and cleanliness became articulated with the growing social science discourses with the founding of the Ladies' National Association for the Diffusion of Sanitary Knowledge in 1857. This was a sub-group of the Association for the Promotion of Social Science, which had been founded one year earlier and, unusually for that time, admitted women as full members. This Association continued to express concern about the hygienic circumstances in which the working class lived and about the ignorance of mothers. Attention was particularly drawn to the fatal effects in poor districts of childhood and infant diarrhoea, whooping cough, measles and bronchitis, illnesses that were seldom fatal among middle- and upper-class children. It tended to be suggested that the excessive infant mortality rate was mainly due to the ill management of children by their parents.

The Ladies' Sanitary Association set up branches around the country. Like the Visiting Societies they visited the homes of the poor on a systematic basis, but they were specifically concerned to distribute information on matters of health. There is some dispute as to when the first 'health visitors' (as they were later called) were employed. Many accounts (e.g. Dingwall, 1979; McCleary, 1933) argue that it was in Manchester in 1867; however, Dowling (1963) suggests that when the Manchester Ladies' Sanitary Association was formed there were already 134 woman Bible/sanitary missionaries employed in London. Certainly Mrs Raynor, a founding member of the Association in London, was the first person to employ a working-class woman to visit the homes of the poor disseminating religious tracts and giving advice on matters of hygiene. However, the title 'health (sanitary) visitor' was first used in Manchester, and Manchester Corporation was the first to take on the responsibility for paying salaries to health visitors, in 1890 — although by that time some local authorities were employing lady sanitary inspectors (Dowling, 1963). During the second half of the nineteenth century a number of branches of the Ladies' Sanitary Association were founded, mainly in large towns. Generally working-class women were paid from charitable monies to visit the homes of the poor, but they were supervised by unpaid middle-class women. Initially the working-class visitors had been untrained, but by the end of the nineteenth century there were some moves towards providing training. (For a detailed history see Dowling, 1963.)

By the end of the nineteenth century, then, we have a relatively small number of employed working-class women visiting the homes of the poor. Their geographical distribution was also uneven. The work of these women was supervised by middle-class volunteers. Although the Sanitary Reform Movement and the sanitary reform legislation demonstrated some recognition that health and hygiene were at the mercy of factors beyond the control of individuals, the sanitary visiting movement clearly had an individualistic approach. The problem was seen as the neglect by the working class of matters of hygiene and cleanliness, and the solution as the instruction of the poor (and especially poor women). The movement was heavily dominated by *laissez-faire* ideas and much constrained by the reluctance of the state to tax citizens to pay for reforms and improve the conditions of the poor.

Health Visiting in the Twentieth Century

In the early twentieth century, however, in response to what were perceived as 'new' dangers to the health of the British population, health visiting began to develop more rapidly and health visitors became agents in the construction of the 'new' working-class mother.[6] The new concerns provided the space to justify intervention in the family and to overcome the view that children were the property of their parents alone; medical discourses and the developing discourses of psychology provided the 'knowledge' with which to justify and on which to base the form that the interventions took.

In the first decade of the twentieth century there developed a growing concern about the health and fitness of the population; Weeks (1981) has suggested that it amounted to a moral panic. This concern was informed by the two scientific discourses of eugenics and neo-hygienism; that is, these discourses identified/created the problem, targeted certain groups or individuals as the 'cause' of it and suggested strategies of intervention to 'solve' it. One of the key figures created and targeted in the debate was 'the neglectful mother', and of specific concern was the working-class mother who did not provide a hygienic environment for her children and who was seen as even more neglectful if she went out to work. The neglect was seen as the outcome of poor domestic management rather than of poverty or the conditions in which the poor lived. These assumptions about working and neglectful mothers shaped the early infant welfare services. Furthermore, it became accepted that the regulation of the quality of the population was a proper concern of the state, that the conditions of urban life were deleterious to the health and well-being of the working class, that pathological physical and moral states were hereditable and that there was evidence of the progressive degeneration of the population (see Abbott, 1982; Abbott and Sapsford, 1987). It became accepted that the population was something to be valued, known and categorized and that the state could and should play a key role in surveying and monitoring its health.

These developments marked a transition from nineteenth-century *laissez-faire* attitudes to poverty. In the nineteenth century the individual was seen as responsible for his or her own poverty and unfitness. Pauperism was seen as the result of individual failure, and the pauper as needing to be regulated and controlled — the problem was the poor, not poverty. There had been some concern over the conditions created by urbanization, resulting in reform of insanitary conditions as a means of improving the health of the (working-class) population as well as the 'sanitary visiting' movements to which we have referred. The surveys of Booth (1890) and Rowntree (1901) into urban poverty and pauperism, however, had a substantial impact on thinking about poverty and its causes. Booth argued that it was necessary to make a clear distinction between the employable and unemployable poor. Not all poverty could be blamed on the moral and physical characteristics of those living in it. Unemployment could then be seen as both the cause of poverty (for the employable) and the outcome of their own nature (for the unemployable). This enabled a distinction to be drawn between members of society (the employable) and those considered unemployable who should therefore be excluded from society.

The science of eugenics (influenced by social Darwinism) argued that anti-social behaviour was an inherited characteristic and that the race was degenerating in this respect. In the nineteenth century it had been accepted that acquired characteristics could be inherited and therefore that improvement in the population could be brought about by environmental reform (see Abbott, 1982; Abbott and Sapsford, 1987) — although the dominant *laissez-faire* view was that the state should not intervene in poverty but allow the proper laws of nature to function so that the unfit died out. However, the eugenicists accepted Weissman's view that acquired traits could not be inherited. The rediscovered work of Mendel armed them with a possible key for developing programmes of planned propagation. The eugenicists, and particularly Galton, Pearson and White, argued that there was a scientific basis for explaining the degeneration of the British race and for planning programmes to remedy it. Racial progress would come from the scientific control of nature — from preventing tainted stock from propagating. This meant that the norm had to be established scientifically and scientific methods of singling out the unfit developed. In 1901 Galton argued that he had found a link between population variation and norm, human heredity, and the problem of urban degeneracy. Booth, he pointed out, had divided the population into a number of classes, and he argued that the distribution of and numbers in these classes followed the pattern that would have been predicted by the normal laws of frequency (see his Huxley Lecture to the Anthropological Institute in October of 1901). The influence of the eugenics movement in the early twentieth century is disputed (compare Rose, 1985, with Weeks, 1981). We would suggest that apart from being a determining influence on the 'problem' of the feeble-minded it also focused attention on 'racial degeneration' and led to the development and use of intelligence tests to separate the fit from the unfit — a practice that persists in much scientific and common-sense thought to this day and results in a considerable amount of routine testing, including the age-normed developmental tests routinely carried out by health visitors.

The discourse of eugenics articulated with imperialist discourses in the late nineteenth century — with a growing concern about Britain's position as a leading world power. Concern grew that the population was deteriorating physically and psychologically at the same time as it seemed that Britain was declining as a military, industrial and commercial nation. The economic recession of the 1870s, the defeat of Gordon at Khartoum at the hands of 'natives', the debates surrounding the Contagious Diseases Act and the military and industrial growth of Germany and the United States all fanned the fires of concern. At the time of the Boer War (1889–1902) these fears were heightened by the 'discovery' that so many of the enlisted men had to be discharged as unfit after a short period of service. In the medical journals and other publications, medical men and eugenicists voiced their concern about the poor state of health of the British population and the possibility of progressive degeneracy. This concern, that the physical and mental quality of the population was declining, was increased by class-specific differential birth-rates. While the middle class (and even the respectable working class) had reduced the size of their families during the late nineteenth century, the lower working class (the disreputable and unemployable) were still having large families. In other words, according to the eugenicists, the unfit were outbreeding the fit. Eugenic methods were necessary either to encourage the fit to breed or to prevent the unfit from doing so.

At the same time a different concern about the health of the population was being articulated. During the nineteenth century, presumably as a consequence of sanitary reform and improvement in housing and diet (McKeown, 1976), the life expectancy of the population had risen. However, during the last decade of the century concern grew about the infant mortality rate, which had not only not declined along with the general mortality rate but in some years actually went up. Although a number of causes of infant death were acknowledged, attention focused on summer diarrhoea for two main reasons: it was seen as preventable, and it attacked and killed healthy as well as sickly children and could therefore not be seen as eugenic in the way that, for example, wasting diseases might be. While the eugenicists had argued that sanitary reforms, poor law reforms, etc., enabled the genetically unfit to survive and reproduce, the medical discourses surrounding infantile diarrhoea did highlight environmental conditions. However, neo-hygienists focused on hygiene in the home and methods of infant care, including feeding. Mothers were seen as the main cause of infant death and by implication of poor health in children and adults (see, e.g., Black, 1915; Rathbone, 1924; Bell, 1907).[7]

As a consequence of the fears about the health of the population, an Interdepartmental Committee on Physical Deterioration was set up, and it reported in 1904. The Committee heard from a wide range of experts but carried out no original research. It rejected the eugenicist arguments and accepted environmentalist and hygienist ones. It argued, however, that there was a need to improve the health of children and accepted the evidence put to it that one of the major problems was neglectful and employed working-class mothers. Among a large number of recommendations, it suggested the employment of health visitors. Probably this recommendation was taken up because health visiting was seen as an inexpensive way of dealing with the problem, as opposed to the high cost of improving the housing, environment and wages of the poor.

The environmentalist school, freed from the view that acquired characteristics could become hereditable, focused attention on the household, which was seen as a machine for the raising of children. Mothers were seen as having the main responsibility for rearing a physically, mentally and morally efficient population. The eugenicist movement, however, influenced the debates on mental deficiency, especially feeble-mindedness, and prevailed with the view that it was necessary to monitor the population and segregate the mentally unfit. Rose (1985) has argued that the eugenicist and neo-hygienist strategies (i.e. strategies aimed at teaching knowledge of hygiene, not just changing the environment) became combined in a single scheme of administration — a programme that was concerned to differentiate between the socializable and the residuum, the former subject to a regime of benevolent improvement, medical scrutiny and education, the latter to segregation. The Mental Deficiency Act 1913, with its provisions for the life-long segregation of the feeble-minded, was the major achievement of the eugenicist movement (Weeks, 1981; Abbott, 1982; Abbott and Sapsford, 1987).

The neo-hygienists had much more impact on welfare measures in the early twentieth century and on the health education directed at mothers. They translated concern about public health into individualistic preventive medicine which targeted especially the working-class mother. While in the first decade of the century attention was focused on the neglectful mother and especially on infant feeding practices — contamination being seen as a major cause of infantile diarrhoea — by the end of the First World War the concern had widened to include the health of the mother as well as that of the child (Rowan, 1985). The work of the Women's Co-operative Guild in collating the letters of women on maternity and the realization that the health of women and children improved while men were away at war and the women were dependent on war allowances (Rowan, 1984) helped in this process. Nevertheless, while health was seen as something positive and to be sought, its achievement was thought to be brought about by scrutinizing individuals and the relationships between them at the level of the family. The key figure was the mother, who, it was argued, was responsible for the health of her family. The target of intervention was therefore the mother; effort was directed at training her as a mother and inspecting the home, the inspection of infants and school-children and the provision of school meals for needy children. However, despite the concern for children, they were excluded from the National Insurance Act 1911, and infant welfare centres and school doctors could only inspect children, not treat them. While families and especially mothers, it was argued, were to bring up their children on behalf of the nation, and the state had a right and a duty to ascertain that they were doing this, it was the family that remained responsible for providing for the medical and other needs of their children. (While the Campaign for the Endowment of Motherhood dates from this period, it was not until 1976 that mothers received the total amount of state financial support for their children with the abolition of child tax allowances in favour of an allowance paid to the mother. In recent years public policy has tended to move away from the endowment of motherhood and back towards a means-tested provision based on total family income — see Dominelli, 1988.)

The bulwark of the infant welfare movement was the health visitor. The title used to refer to these workers was itself important. Many of the early workers in the field had been employed as sanitary inspectors, but the term 'health visitor' was preferred because it did not carry overtones of inspection. Florence Nightingale described the health visitor's role as helping the mother and making no judgments, and Sir Thomas Barlow stressed that the health visitor was not to be regarded as a policeman or sanitary inspector (see Greenwood, 1913). The importance of being non-judgmental was also reinforced by health visitors themselves in the evidence they gave to the 1904 Interdepartmental Committee. Whether employed by a local authority or a voluntary organization, health visitors visited the working-class mother in her home to advise on hygiene and infant care and management as well as to inspect the home. They were also employed by the milk kitchens and schools for mothers and by the infant welfare clinics. In this period not only did their numbers grow, but the occupation was transformed. The state became increasingly involved with the work of health visiting. An increasing number of local authorities began to employ health visitors (who worked under the direction of the medical officer of health); the Notification of Births Act 1909 (made mandatory in 1915) was designed so that health visitors could visit all new-born babies as soon after birth as possible, and central government not only suggested that local authorities should employ them but also assisted with funds. In 1917 the Local Government Board stated that all sanitary authorities should employ them and that it had money for grants to aid expenditure in respect of maternity and child welfare services (Local Government Board, 1917).

In its 1917 Report the Local Government Board stressed that the main responsibility of health visitors was to advise mothers on matters of hygiene and infant care. It was suggested that they should visit all mothers as soon after the birth of the baby as possible and certainly by the tenth day. They should also visit cases of ophthalmia neonatorum and young children with certain infectious diseases. In the summer, they should pay calls on all homes with young children to warn against the dangers of epidemic diarrhoea, ensure that any child suffering from it was being properly cared for and look into the death of any child to ascertain the cause of death. It noted that health visitors' duties were being extended to include visiting expectant mothers and by continuing the visitation of infants until they reached school age. Additionally, health visitors were being used at infant welfare clinics. The Board also recognized that the actual provision of health visitors, the duties they undertook and the frequency with which they made visits varied widely throughout the country.

During the period when the state was taking over responsibility for health visiting, the type of person becoming a health visitor also changed. While its status remained low, health visiting became seen as a suitable vocation for middle-class women rather than just a philanthropic endeavour. In the late nineteenth century it had begun to be argued that some training should be provided. Buckingham County Council was the first local authority to provide a training course, in 1892, but it was in the early twentieth century that permanent formal courses as a recognized route to qualification were established, that it became compulsory for employed health visitors to be so qualified, and that health visitors were required to have nursing and midwifery qualifications. In 1907 Bedford College for Women and Battersea Polytechnic started a two-year course for educated women (and a six-month course for trained nurses), so the link between health visiting and nursing was not yet a necessary one. In 1908 the Royal Sanitary Institute started to set a health visiting examination. (It remained the examining body until the establishment of the Council for the Education and Training of Health Visitors in 1965, now itself replaced by the National Nursing Board.) In 1909 London County Council laid down that in future all its health visitors should have a medical degree, full nurse training or a certificate of the Central Board of Midwives, have been previously employed as a health visitor or else have some nurse training and a Health Visitor's Certificate. In 1916 the Local Government Board recommended that health visitors should have two of three qualifications: nurse training, a Sanitary Inspector's Certificate or a Certificate of the Central Midwives' Board. In 1919 the Ministry of Health and the Board of Education recommended three modes of entry: a one-year post-nursing course, a different one-year course for university graduates, or a two-year course for others. In 1925 the Ministry of Health required that all new entrants have midwifery training, and in 1928 that they have a Health Visitor's Certificate. Subsequently the period of training was reduced to six months for nurses (but increased again to a year in 1965), and the courses for people other than nurses died out because they failed to attract students. (However, it was not until 1962 that SRN certification became a requirement for entry to training.)

By the 1920s health visiting had become firmly established as a state service employing low-status semi-professional female workers, working under the direction of doctors (medical officers of health). The health visitor's main role was educating mothers in the care of young children, monitoring child development and inspecting the homes of the working class. By the 1930s, with the infant mortality rate declining, there was a move towards greater emphasis on child care — improving the health of surviving children (McCleary, 1933). Health visitors came increasingly to be seen as well baby nurses. Their knowledge/power was based on neo-hygienic/medical discourses on the causes of ill health and especially infant diarrhoea, but underpinned by eugenic ideas of separating the fit from the unfit. In this role they played a largely symbolic role in constructing and policing the 'new mother' — the woman whose main responsibility was ensuring the physical, mental and moral health of her children (and husband) on behalf of the nation. The intervention of the state's representatives in the family was legitimated by concern about national efficiency. Child protection was justified while health visitors could claim to be helping mothers to achieve what they wanted — the best for their children. Health visitors played a role in creating and identifying the 'inadequate mother'. They then became involved in programmes of reform to transform her, to shape her behaviour so that she becomes an adequate, a 'good enough' mother.

While advice on hygiene continues to be one of the functions of the health visitor, work with families has widened to include advice on the mental, emotional and cognitive development of children. Health visitors have also become more aware of the societal causes of social problems, although their interventions still tend to be individualistic. Events in the 1930s and the experience of widespread unemployment dissolved, if only temporarily, the linkage between personal characteristics and unemployment and between personal habits and social problems. It was recognized that social problems were located in society rather than in the individual. This resulted in the acceptance of the right of citizenship — that everyone should enjoy fundamental basic rights — and the acceptance also of the idea that the state should intervene to plan economic activity and social services. In the same period doctors and nutritionalists began to show the relationship between income, diet and health, and this gave further impetus to the campaign for the endowment of motherhood. Thus the space was created for discourses that saw material differences as the main problem to be solved. The welfare legislation after the Second World War was designed to eradicate poverty and provide adequate health care for all citizens, while the associated management of the economy was to ensure full employment. Social workers were to pick up the casualties of the welfare state — those who could not cope without additional support. Health visiting, however, became a universal service, concerned with monitoring the health of the whole population, but with a major responsibility still for the pre-school child and his or her family. A need was still seen to reduce infant and child mortality further and to improve the health of children. In this period, as after World War I, there was concern about a decline in the size of the population. As we have noted already, while the discourses may have emphasized the importance of the family as a unit, in practice health visiting intervention continued to target the mother and to be concerned with the health and development of young children.

Health visitors continued to play a major role in the surveillance of the family and in 'creating' mothers, especially in a period when the 'need' for mothers to work full time in the home was being stressed (Riley, 1983). Their knowledge had come to incorporate new discourses on mental health which argued that major mental disturbances were preventable by early recognition and treatment. Part of the health visitors' role became the surveillance of *mental* hygiene, to pick up minor problems before they developed into major ones. They also incorporated new ideological propositions influenced by Freudian theory — propositions which stressed that the natural family was a biological necessity for the healthy development of the children, that it provided the right environment for the development of a harmonious and well rounded character. Increasingly mothers began to be held responsible not just for the health of their children but for their emotional and cognitive development, which gave them responsibility for (and the experts a legitimate concern with) children's day-to-day thoughts and feelings. Thus health visitors began to work with the 'knowledge' that particular familial relations were correct/desirable. After World War II the work of Bowlby and Winnicott came to dominate ideas on children, and especially ideas on the role of the mother as the key figure in the normal development of children. Bonding became a key concept in the work of health visitors, who stressed the important role that mothers played in the development of their children and the young child's need for mothering by a loving, natural mother. (Thus mothers became responsible to health visitors and other experts for the nature of their feelings towards their children.) The Jameson Report emphasized that health visitors were likely to be increasingly concerned with the mental aspects of health, especially as the need for advice on physical aspects was declining. Especially important would be advice on the importance of a normal and happy family life for the mental health of the child. (So the mother was responsible to the health visitor even for whether she was happy or not.) This change in emphasis was reflected in the new syllabus for health visitor training introduced in 1965.

Conclusions

A history of health visiting enables us to see that the confusions and ambiguities that confront health visitors are rooted in their origins and development. A number of discourses have informed health visiting and continue to inform it — medical/sanitary, philanthropic, psychological/psychiatric — and it is shaped by and plays its role as agent of social control through a number of not always compatible ideological positions. To all this is added the ambiguity of the professional status of health visitors and the concern over their identity as nurses. We can see, then, why they are uncertain about their precise role, scope and status. With reduction in infant mortality rates and improvement in the diet, housing and environment of a majority of the population the need for them to advise mothers on how to keep their children alive has decreased, and with it their original *raison d'être*. They have moved into the 'child development business', where they have become the main workers because they see every child at an early age, but this is an area already well colonized by people with better paper claims to expertise, such as psychologists, psychiatrists and pediatricians. The uncertainty of the relationship between health visiting, nursing and social work and the lack of a clear and distinctive knowledge base for health visiting are also explicable by the way in which health visiting has grown and changed, particularly during the twentieth century. Health visitors' individualistic mode of intervention, paralleling that of medicine and social work, has been challenged by cultural and political/economic explanations for health inequalities, as well as by the feminist movement. The low status of health visiting and the medical dominance over its practice is clearly rooted in the importance of medical discourse in its foundation and development. Like nurses, health visitors were in part established to work on behalf of and under the direction of medical men (or, in the very early years, under lady volunteers who themselves accepted the advice and direction of medical men). The problems they experience in extricating themselves from this dominance and establishing an independent professional status relate to the development of health visiting as a female occupation based on medical knowledge at a time when medical knowledge was a male preserve.

The critique of social workers, from both the left and the right, as agents of social control interested in furthering their own professional status at the expense of working-class clients, has also caused health visitors to examine their own mode of intervention in the family. This examination is also a result of increased emphasis on visibly providing value for money, of demonstrating the value of the service and of increased accountability — difficult for a service whose traditional role has been universal monitoring, with the expectation that active intervention will very seldom be required. The question of selectivity versus universalism has been a key issue in recent development. Health visiting started as a selective intervention (into the lives of working-class women) but has become a universal one under the influence of discourse which creates emotional/cognitive development as a prime object of attention and posits it as something not necessarily less likely to be problematic in middle-class than in working-class homes. Health visitors feel it necessary to justify their surveillance of all families with young children — that all mothers need advice and education in child care, that it is as necessary to monitor psychological as physical development, and that cruelty and neglect can be psychological as well as physical. (The evidence now suggests that physical cruelty and sexual abuse towards children may not be less common in middle-class than in working-class homes, but this tends to pose a problem for health visitors rather than provide a justification for them, as they retain — if only on pragmatic grounds — their original emphasis on non-coercive work with and on behalf of the mother rather than against her on behalf of the state or even the child.)

It seems to us that while there continues to be strong support for the view that poor health is the result of individual inadequacies and widespread support also for the view that children need protecting, there will continue to be support for a health visiting service. However, if the Thatcher Government continues with neo-liberal policies in the health and welfare services then health visiting in the form in which it exists at present will be forced into radical change, to become more selective, to deal with a wider group of client types and to be more accountable for its day-to-day practice. If the recommendations of recent nursing reports are accepted and the National Nursing Board continues to dominate the debates then health visitors will become more clearly identified with nurses and more closely supervised. While they may become more highly qualified, they will work within a more bureaucratic structure and have less control over their work — that is, they will become de-skilled. Given this, one may doubt whether they will become recognized by doctors as professionals of equal standing, and they will remain under medical dominance.

Finally, we should return to the question with which this chapter opened: are health visitors social policemen? Clearly they have attempted to develop a non-judgmental style of work and to concentrate on developing good relationships with clients. They have none of the legal powers of social workers or doctors, nor any control over financial resources, nor do they have a legal right of entry into the home. The advice that they give does not have to be heeded, and there is very little they can do to change the behaviour of individuals or families who resist their advice. Despite all this, they do attempt to shape the behaviour of individuals, to encourage them to conform to societal norms. They work with certain assumptions of what these norms are, and their individualistic mode of intervention encourages the notion that problems can be solved at that level. Education, as we have said, is not neutral; it embodies values and attitudes which may not initially be shared by those being educated. The process of education in this context means the setting of priorities and, by teaching the means of attaining child welfare, the reinforcement of the notion that the child's welfare outweighs that of the parents. Working almost entirely with women, health visitors help to ensure that it is *mothers* on whom this burden falls, and so they unwittingly reinforce the necessity of a service role for women. This is not to deny that health visitors do help those with whom they work. Nevertheless it does mean that they act to some extent as agents of social control, reinforcing societal norms and disseminating individualistic explanations for social problems. This is the case even if they themselves recognize the social/economic causes of these problems, because of the individualistic mode of their interaction. Indeed, while we have stressed in this chapter that health visitors are confused about their role, few of them seem to experience any ambiguity surrounding their non-judgmental stance. This, we would suggest, is because they are not themselves aware of the ways in which they police the family: they accept as 'truth' the discourses that inform their practice and therefore fail to recognize the ways in which they are used to shape the behaviour of clients.

Notes

1. To avoid confusions and the possibility of identifying particular informants to whom we have referred in this text, health visitors are described as female throughout the chapter. The vast majority of health visitors are indeed women: men became able to enter training only when changed legislation enabled them to undertake obstetric training.
2. The Cumberledge Report: this was the report of an inquiry into community nursing. It recommended the establishment of community nursing teams based on geographical areas. It expressed the hope that GPs could move to being responsible for the population of a geographical area, thus enabling primary health care teams to be established. In the absence of this change it argued for the nursing team to be geographically based even if the nursing area did not map on to doctors' practices. The

response of the BMA and the Government suggests that it is unlikely that GPs will become geographically based.

3. The Health Visiting Process is the adaptation to health visiting of the Nursing Process. This in turn is a problem-oriented approach to nursing. It assumes that nursing is based on a systematic body of knowledge which can be used to solve or alleviate the problems of individual patients. It involves the nurse in assessiang a patient's needs and identifying the problems that can be helped by nursing intervention, developing a programme of care and monitoring and evaluating the outcome (see Rogers, 1982; Clarke, 1980, 1982).

4. *Nursing 2000* was a report on the future of nurse training. One of its main recommendations was that there should be one common basic qualification, but with more specialist post-registration courses. It also argued that the title 'nurse' should be reserved for qualified nurses and that nursing auxiliaries and other non-qualified nurses should be referred to as aides. The training provisions are now in process of implementation.

5. We are acutely aware of the criticisms that can be made of Foucault's work, and especially the charges of social constructionism and relativism (see, for example, Bury, 1986; Nicolson and McLaughlin, 1987; Turner, 1987). We are not arguing that Foucault has provided a new theory/methodology for sociological analysis, and we specifically reject the view that he has demonstrated that modes of information have replaced modes of production as an explanation for social change (Smart, 1985). Indeed, we have argued elsewhere that it is socio-economic changes that produce the conditions under which discourses become thinkable and implementable (Abbott and Sapsford, 1988 — and see also Cohen, 1985).

6. Familial ideology in the nineteenth century had already established the idea that women and children should be dependent on men and that men should be paid a 'family wage'. Certainly by the beginning of the twentieth century this idea was firmly established (see, e.g., Roberts, 1984). Also, in the nineteenth century middle-class women had become identified as principally wives and mothers responsible for the care of their children (but see Helterine, 1980). What was new about the early twentieth century was that women came to be seen as guardians of their children on behalf of the nation. (This of course enabled women to fight back and demand some payment for carrying out this responsibility.)

7. While these feminist accounts clearly document the dominant identification of the neglectful mother, they also clearly argue that the major problem was poverty. They demonstrate vividly how women managed to raise large families in constant poverty and themselves suffering poor health. While they recognize that some women were better managers than others, they document that these were 'superwomen', not a norm which other women should be 'fired' to imitate. Indeed, reading these accounts one is left to marvel at how anyone could manage to feed and care for a family on the incomes of many households. There are also indications, though not much firm evidence, that working-class women resented the advice and interference of health visitors (see, e.g., Thane, 1982).

References

ABBOTT, P. A. (1982) *Towards a Social Theory of Mental Handicap*, Ph.D. thesis, Thames Polytechnic.

ABBOTT, P. A. and SAPSFORD, R. J. (1987) *'Community Care' for Mentally Handicapped Children: the origins and consequences of a social policy*, Milton Keynes, Open University Press.

ABBOTT, P. A. and SAPSFORD, R. J. (1988) 'The Body Politic: health, family and society', Unit 11 of Open University course D211 *Social Problems and Social Welfare*, Milton Keynes, The Open University.

BANKS, O. (1981) *Faces of Feminism*, Oxford, Martin Robertson.

BELL, LADY (1907) *At the Works*, republished, with an introduction by A. V. Johns, London, Virago, 1983.

BELLIS, G. (1981) 'The primary health care team', *Health Visitor*, **54**, May, p. 188.

BENNETT, E. M. (1918) 'Babies in peril', *Maternity and Child Welfare*, **2**, November, pp. 370–76; and **2**, December, pp. 410–18.

BLACK, C. (Ed.) (1915) *Married Women's Work*, republished, with an introduction by E. Mappen, London, Virago, 1983.

BLAND, L. and MORT, C. (1984) 'Look out for the "good time" girl', in *Formation of Nation and People*, London, Routledge and Kegan Paul.

BOOTH, W. (1890) *In Darkest England and the Way Out*, London.

BRISCOE, M. and LINDLEY, P. (1982) 'Identification and management of psychological problems by health visitors', *Health Visitor*, **55**, April, pp. 165–9.

BRIGGS REPORT (1972) *Report of the Committee on Nursing*, London, HMSO.

BURY, M. R. (1986) 'Social constructionism and the development of medical sociology', *Sociology of Health and Illness*, **8**, pp. 137–69.

CARTLIDGE, A. M. (1985) *Perceptions of Teamwork in Primary Health Care Organisations*, Newcastle, University of Newcastle Health Care Research Unit.

CHADWICK, E. (1842) *Report on the Sanitary Conditions of the Labouring Population of Great Britain*, republished, with an introduction by M. W. Flein, Edinburgh, Edinburgh University Press, 1965.

CLARKE, JOHN (1988) 'Social work: the personal and the political', Unit 13 of Open University course D211 *Social Problems and Social Welfare*, Milton Keynes, The Open University.

CLARKE, JUNE (1970) *The Health Visitor's Point of View*, paper presented to the Health Congress of the Royal Society of Health, Eastbourne.

CLARKE, JUNE (1972) 'The "new bred" health visitor', *Nursing Times*, **68**, 31, pp. 121–2.

CLARKE, JUNE (1980) 'A framework for health visiting: a systems approach', Part I: 'The application of systems theory to health visiting', *Health Visitor*, **53**, October, pp. 419–21; Part II: 'The nature of health visiting activity', *Health Visitor*, **53**, November, pp. 487–535.

CLARKE, JUNE (1982) 'A way to get organised', *Nursing Times*, 15 October, pp. 287–97.

COHEN, S. (1985) *Visions of Social Control*, Cambridge, Polity.

COURT REPORT (1976) *Fit for the Future: Report of the Committee on the Child Health Services*, Cmnd. 6684, London, HMSO.

CUMBERLEDGE REPORT (1986) *Neighbourhood Nursing: a focus for care*, London, HMSO.

DAVID, M. E. (1985) 'Motherhood and social policy — a matter of education?', *Critical Social Policy*, **12**, pp. 28–43.

DAVIN, A. (1978) 'Imperialism and motherhood', *History Workshop*, 5, pp. 9–63.

DEATH, E. (1982) 'A preventive approach to family life: the role of the health visitor', *Health Visitor*, 55, June, pp. 282–4.

DINGWALL, R. (1979) *The Social Organisation of Health Visiting*, Beckenham, Croom Helm.

DINGWALL, R. (1982) 'Community nursing and civil liberty', *Journal of Advanced Nursing*, 7, pp. 337–46.

DOMINELLI, L. (1988) 'Thatcher's attack on social security: restructuring social control', *Critical Social Policy*, 23, pp. 46–61.

DONZELOT, J. (1977) *The Policing of Families*, London, Hutchinson, 1980.

DOWLING, W. G. (1963) *The Ladies' Sanitary Association and the Origins of the Health Visiting Service*, MA thesis, University of London.

DRAPER, J. *et al.* (1984) 'The working relationship between the general practitioner and the health visitor', *Journal of the Royal College of General Practitioners*, May.

FOUCAULT, M. (1975) *Discipline and Punish: the birth of the prison*, Harmondsworth, Allen Lane, 1977.

FOUCAULT, M. (1976) *The History of Sexuality Vol. I: an introduction*, Harmondsworth, Allen Lane, 1979.

GREENWOOD, F. J. (1913) 'The evolution of the health visitor', *Journal of the Royal Sanitary Institute*, 34, pp. 174–82.

HEALTH VISITORS' ASSOCIATION (undated —a) *Health Visiting: a manifesto*, London, HVA.

HEALTH VISITORS' ASSOCIATION (undated —b) *Health Visiting in the 80s*, London, HVA.

HEARN, J. (1982) 'Notes on patriarchy, professionalisation and the semi-professional', *Sociology*, 16, pp. 184–202.

HELTERINE, M. (1980) 'The emergence of modern motherhood: motherhood in England 1899–1959', *International Journal of Women's Studies*, 3, pp. 590–614.

HEWITT, M. (1983) 'Biopolitics and social policy: Foucault's account of welfare', *Theory, Culture and Society*, 2, pp. 67–84.

HILL, C. (1971) 'The role conflict of the new breed health visitor', *Health Visitor*, 44, pp. 120–22.

HUNT, M. (1977) 'The dilemma of identity in health visiting', *Nursing Times*, 2 February, pp. 17–20; and 10 February, pp. 22–4.

JAMESON REPORT (1956) *An Enquiry into Health Visiting*, London, HMSO.

JEFFERYS, M. (1965) *An Anatomy of Social Welfare Services*, London, Michael Joseph.

LOCAL GOVERNMENT BOARD (1917) *Maternity and Child Welfare*, London, HMSO.

MCCLEARY, G. P. (1933) *The Early History of the Infant Welfare Movement*, London, H. K. Lewis.

MCKEOWN, T. (1976) *The Role of Medicine: dream, mirage or nemesis?*, London, Nuffield Hospital Trust.

MACQUEEN, I. A. G. (1962) 'From carbolic powder to social counsel', *Nursing Times*, 6 July, pp. 866–8.

MANCHESTER HEALTH SOCIETY (1893) *The Ladies' Health Society of Manchester and Salford*, Manchester, Richard Bell.

MEERABEAU, L. (1982) 'Improving the image', *Health Visitor*, 55, June, pp. 298–9.

NEWMAN, G. (1906) *Infant Mortality: a social problem*, London, Methuen.

NICOLSON, N. and MCLAUGHLIN, C. (1987) 'Social constructionism and medical sociology: a reply to M. R. Bury', *Sociology of Health and Illness*, 9, pp. 107–26.

OAKLEY, A. (1984) 'The importance of being a nurse', *Nursing Times*, 12 December, pp. 24–7.

ORR, J. (1986) 'Feminism and health visiting', in WEBB, C. (Ed.) *Feminist Practice in Women's Health Care*, Chichester, Wiley.

PARTON, N. (1985) *The Politics of Child Abuse*, London, Macmillan.

PROCKOSKA, F. K. (1980) *Women and Philanthropy in Nineteenth Century England*, Oxford, Clarendon.

RATHBONE, E. (1924) *The Disinherited Family*, republished, with an introduction by S. Fleming, London, Falling Wall Press, 1986.

RIGLER, M. (1982) 'Tomorrow's health visitor: can she change our attitudes to health?', *Health Visitor*, 55, March, pp. 107–8.

RILEY, D. (1983) *War in the Nursery: theories of the child and mother*, London, Virago.

ROBERTS, E. (1984) *Women in England: sexual division and social change 1870-1950*, Brighton, Wheatsheaf.

ROBINSON, G. (1849) *On Education as Connected with the Sanitary Movement in Newcastle*, London, Longmans.

ROBINSON, J. (1980) *An Evaluation of Health Visiting*, London, CETHV.

ROBINSON, J. (1985) 'Health visiting and health', in WHITE, A. (Ed.) *Political Issues in Nursing: past, present and future Vol. I*, Chichester, Wiley.

ROGERS, J. (1982) 'Introducing the Health Visiting Process', *Health Visitor*, 55, May, pp. 204–9.

ROSE, N. (1985) *The Psychology Complex: psychology, politics and society in England 1869-1939*, London, Routledge and Kegan Paul.

ROSE, N. (1989) 'Individualising psychology', in SHOTTER, J. and GERGEN, K. J. (Eds) *Texts of Identity*, London, Sage.

ROWAN, C. (1984) 'For the duration only: motherhood and nation in the First World War', in *Formation of Nation and People*, London, Routledge and Kegan Paul.

ROWAN, C. (1985) 'Child welfare and the working-class family', in LANGAN, M. and SCHWARZ, B. (Eds) *Crisis in the British State 1880-1930*, London, Hutchinson.

ROWNTREE, B. S. (1901) *Poverty: a study of town life*, London, Macmillan.

ROYAL COLLEGE OF NURSING (1971) *Report of the Working Party on the Role of the Health Visitor Now and in a Changing National Health Service*, London, RCN.

ROYAL COLLEGE OF NURSING (1983) *Thinking About Health Visiting*, London, RCN.

SACHS, H. (1982) 'Health visitors as other professionals see them', *Health Visitor*, 55, June, pp. 292–5.

SALVAGE, J. (1985) *The Politics of Nursing*, London, Heinemann.

SAPSFORD, R. J. (1990) *Discourse, Ideology and Family*, paper prepared for the annual conference of the British Sociological Association, at Guildford.

SCHROCK, R. (1982) 'Is health visiting a profession?', *Health Visitor*, 55, March, pp. 104–7.

SMART, B. (1985) *Michel Foucault*, London, Tavistock.

THANE, P. (1982) *Foundations of the Welfare State*, London, Longmans.

TURNER, B. (1987) *Medical Power and Social Knowledge*, London, Sage.

WARNOCK REPORT (1978) *Special Educational Needs: Report of the Committee of Enquiry into the Education of Handicapped Children and Young People*, London, HMSO.

WEEKS, J. (1981) *Sex, Politics and Society: the regulation of sexuality since 1800*, London, Longmans.

WILSON, M. and COWAN, J. (1982) 'Putting the Health Visiting Process into practice', *Health Visitor*, 55, May, pp. 209–11.

WISE, S. (1985) *Becoming a Feminist Social Worker*, Manchester, Manchester University Department of Sociology, Studies in Sexual Politics No. 6.

WOHL, A. S. (1986) *Endangered Lives: public health in Victorian England*, London, Dent.

10
The Detention of the Mentally Disordered by the Police under Section 136 of the Mental Health Act

Philip Bean

Introduction

In this chapter I want to review some recent research on Section 136 of the 1983 Mental Health Act, i.e. on the way the police make decisions to detain patients in a place of safety. I shall concentrate on research conducted by MIND (National Association for Mental Health) for this is the most relevant for a study of the semi-professions and the most recent also.

The MIND research is in three parts; one (Stage 1) was concerned with evaluating the various places of safety used by the police under that section (Rogers and Faulkner, 1987). The second (Stage 2) is on the action taken by police from the first contact with mentally disordered persons (Rassaby *et al.*, 1989). The third (Stage 3) was on the way the police and psychiatrists view each other: whether they agree on the appropriateness of the respective referrals from the police, on the way they determine the nature of the arrangements, or on the outcome for the patients (Bean *et al.*, 1989; Rogers, 1989).

There are three main reasons for being interested in this form of police activity. First a theoretical one: on the periphery of psychiatry there is a broad network of quasi-psychiatric persons such as the police who serve as a filtering system who regularly, casually or intermittently accept responsibility for treating mental disorder, for referring it to others, or a mixture of both (Schatzman and Strauss, 1966). Questions here have to do with how the police act: what judgments do they make and what are the conceptual thresholds for recognizing mental disturbance? Moreover, how competent are they to make those judgments? Despite the fact that the police have occupied a central position in the management of deviance and the maintenance of social order — a fact which has led to frequent encounters with the mentally disordered — police handling of mentally disordered people has drawn little sociological interest. This chapter is an attempt to remedy that. Second, an interest in the way the police, as semi-professionals, deal with and are dealt with by higher professionals, in this case the psychiatric/medical profession. Often the police emerge as the dominant group when they meet semi-professionals but less so when they meet full blown professionals such as from medicine or law. Why do they then become subordinates and supplicants? In this chapter attempts are made to answer some of these questions. Third, there is a set of questions more down to earth and related to social and public policy. They centre around new forms of community care: with an increase in the discharge of mental patients from hospital and demands for more 'community care', whatever that may mean, will the police become increasingly involved with the mentally disordered? If so, what then should be their tasks, their duties, and how should they work with other occupational groups? Attempts are made to answer some of these questions too.

Section 136 *and the Law*

Section 136 of the 1983 Mental Health Act provides the focus to this study. This section gives the police powers to remove from a public place a person suspected of being mentally disordered. (The powers to remove a person from a 'private place', e.g. the patient's own home, are covered under other sections of the Mental Health Act.)

Section 136

1. If a constable finds in a place to which the public have access a person who appears to him to be suffering from mental disorder and to be in immediate need of care or control the constable may, if he thinks it necessary to do so in the interests of that person or for the protection of other persons, remove that person to a place of safety within the meaning of Section 135 above.
2. A person removed to a place of safety under this section may be detained there for a period not exceeding 72 hours for the purpose of enabling him to be examined by a registered medical practitioner and to be interviewed by an approved social worker and for making necessary arrangements for his treatment and care.

Essentially what Section 136 says is this:

(a) It authorizes the removal from a public place of a person suspected of being mentally disordered;

(b) it does not provide for compulsory detention as such but allows the police to detain a person in order to make the necessary arrangements for his/her treatment and care;

(c) it involves the police taking the person to a place of safety, which may and often does involve a police station and a mental hospital, and

(d) it involves detaining him/her for up to 72 hours so that he/she may be interviewed by a registered medical practitioner and an approved social worker.

On the face of it this section seems straightforward enough. That is, it gives powers to the police to detain a person who is believed to be mentally disordered in a public place, to take that person to a place of safety where he/she can be detained for up to 72 hours in order that he/she be interviewed by a registered medical practitioner and an approved social worker before making the necessary arrangements for further treatment or care. At one extreme the final decision could involve the person being discharged from the place of safety with no further ado, at the other being compulsorily admitted to a mental hospital under another section of the Mental Health Act. This Section completes and tidies up matters. It completes them in the sense that it deals with the mentally disordered in a public place — the other sections of the 1983 Mental Health Act provide powers for detention of patients in private dwellings. And it tidies up matters in that it gives the police powers to manage and control deviance other than when the person breaks the criminal law. One would have thought that would have been the end of the matter. But this is not so.

We can ignore for these purposes a set of questions raised by lawyers about legal definitions (e.g. what constitutes a public place? What would happen if a constable lured a person from a private to a public place and then detained him/her? And what would happen if the police did not detain a person under Section 136 and the person died or injured him/herself or others? See also Bean, 1986). Instead, we can concentrate on other matters such as where professional rivalries exist and ideological positions are asserted and fought over. Consider professional rivalry: some (social workers and psychiatrists) are critical of the police and police powers because they assert the police lack the required professional training and are unable to diagnose mental disorder appropriately. Moreover the police are said to lack certain sensitivities in dealing with the mentally ill. Whether so or not, there is evidence from earlier studies to suggest that the police are indeed efficient sources of referral — if 'efficiency' is defined as producing high levels of agreement between police and psychiatrists about patients to be admitted

(Berry and Orwin, 1966; Kelleher and Copeland, 1972; Mountney *et al.*, 1969; Sims and Symonds, 1975). On the sensitivity of the police no further comment is needed except to add it would be surprising if social workers and psychiatrists had a monopoly of this.

But before entering the debate about the means and types of referrals we need to ask a more basic question: what is the extent of use of Section 136? And as with all such questions there are no clear answers. Figures produced by the DHSS for 1982 show that 1855 persons were so detained and the numbers being detained are increasing (Rogers, 1989). Two points can be made. First, that we must be sceptical about such figures generally, and those for Section 136 are no exception; and, second, that the official use of Section 136 is almost entirely confined to the Metropolitan Districts of London. There are many reasons why this is so, and these need not be considered here except to note that in many areas of England and Wales local arrangements exist which allow the police to detain individuals on a Section 136 order but do not require them to complete the documentation. Hence, such individuals do not appear in the official figures, yet to all intents and purposes have been detained under Section 136. This is not so for London (see also Bean, 1980).

Criticisms of Section 136

Criticisms about the use of Section 136 come from various quarters, other than those mentioned above. Such criticisms tend to be bound up with wider criticisms about the position and activities of the police generally, and about the police's relationship with ethnic minority groups. One can see how the argument unfolds: the Poor Law and the Vagrancy Acts were designed to solve a problem of law and order in the nineteenth century. These laws have now laregly been repealed. The modern equivalent is Section 136, designed, so its critics would have us believe, to act like the Vagrancy Acts and solve the problem of law and order in the twentieth century. This time minority groups are the target, for they have become the modern equivalent of the restive urban working class of the nineteenth century. So, according to this line of argument, the debate about Section 136 becomes tied into a second debate about the relationships between police and minority groups generally, and the fear and distrust these groups express of the police in particular — especially when they are detained in police stations.

Specific criticisms of Section 136 can for these purposes be reduced to two major areas of police practice: the responsibility for detaining the individual, and where the individual should be detained. In the first, the more radical and extreme view is to argue as some do that Section 136 should be abolished. Those favouring such a position do not doubt there are disordered persons in public places, or that they should be detained — though some may. Mostly they say the individual should be taken directly to hospital by medical and ambulance staff without legal or police intervention. Yet that would seem to provide no solution at all; if anything it would compound, aggravate and perhaps exacerbate the problem. It means, in effect, making medical and ambulance staff surrogate police officers with powers of arrest. Would they accept this and would medical and allied staff be prepared to patrol on a twenty-four hour basis? I think not. Would they also be prepared to undertake all that is involved in detaining difficult, aggressive individuals, even if they were granted powers of arrest similar to those given to the police? Again, I think not. Would they also be prepared to see the ambulances as an acceptable place of safety, and what would happen if, after all this, the hospital refused admission? There are, it seems, many good reasons why the police have to be seen as the one group likely to and indeed able to detain people and be the point of first contact for these mentally disordered persons, for they are the only group who agree to act in this way.

There is a more considered argument, less strident and, I think, more worthy of examination although it too has serious defects: that is, the police should retain their existing powers but as soon as possible thereafter hand the patient over to others such as medical and ambulance staff who would then transfer and hold the individual in a place of safety — always a hospital, never a police station. Contact between police and patients would therefore be reduced. Supposedly, this would benefit certain minority groups and help reduce racial tension: the argument hinges on a wish of minority groups to avoid contact with the police or minimize it as far as possible. I respect these views yet, at the same time, this type of proposal is not without certain practical difficulties. Again, it is not clear if medical and ambulance staff would wish to take on these extra duties. Moreover, the argument contains an assumption which is difficult to accept, that certain political and social problems can be reduced or eradicated if they are medicalized. It is an assumption based on the view that the police are the only occupational group which is prejudiced, or rather that they are more prejudiced than medical and allied staff. It implies that medicalizing a problem reduces conflict and tension. Yet medical and allied staff do not have unblemished records in matters of prejudice. Moreover, conflicts or prejudice are not necessarily reduced under a medical canopy; often they reappear in more covert forms. When such conflict or prejudice exists it is no less easy to resolve, being sustained by structural features linked to professional attitudes and reinforced by institutional supports.

The second area for suggested reform concerns the place of safety itself, that is the place where the individual should be so detained. The police have been advised by the Home Office (see Home Office, 1975, Appendix 7) that a person who is removed under this section should normally be taken direct to a hospital or, if this is not practicable, that the assistance of a social worker should be sought immediately. The duties of the social worker in this are, according to the Butler Report (Butler Report, 1975, para. 9.1):

> contacting the detained person's relatives and ascertaining whether there is a history of psychiatric treatment. Should admission to hospital prove necessary such information gathered by the social worker may indicate which hospital would be most suitable; but the social worker and to some extent the medical practitioner should always consider whether any course other than admission to hospital is appropriate. Knowing the range of resources which is available the social worker is in a position to assess all the circumstances and is responsible for making sure whether treatment in hospital is the only solution.

In spite of such a strong recommendation, or perhaps because of practical difficulties, things do not work quite like that. No one is sure how often the police use the police station as a place of safety, for they are not required to provide this information — and as will be shown later social workers are rarely used. It is suspected, however, that the advice given in the Home Office circular may not often be taken and a police station is used frequently. One can see why. The police may regard the individual as too aggressive or disturbed and may wish to keep their options open and charge the individual with an offence if he is not admitted to a hospital. The police station is more appropriate under these circumstances. Moreover, the social worker is not always the first to be called. The police have to gauge the likely social work and medical response and they may well regard the police station as offering them the best and more predictable form of control.

If the person is not removed to a hospital as recommended by the Home Office and goes to a police station as a place of safety, what are the problems then? One solution suggested is for purpose-built institutions to be provided, staffed and controlled by local authorities. There is no objection to this in principle, assuming that local authorities were prepared to provide such facilities, though they may be less than enthusiastic about taking on such a task. It would be expensive and would mean making their employees custodians with powers of detention and liability to be sued for negligence when it occurred. However, there would be no legal difficulty for such powers already exist. Section 137 (2) says that:

> Any other person authorised by or by virtue of this act to take into custody or to convey or detain any person shall, for the purpose of taking him into custody or conveying him, have all the powers, authorities, protection or privileges which a constable has within the area for which he acts as constable.

And Section 137 (1) says that when a person is so detained he shall be deemed to be in legal custody with all that means in terms of powers granted to those who have to retake those who escape, etc. (Section 138). Such objections as there are may well be on financial, social and moral grounds.

Yet there is another assumption contained in these suggestions: that the individual would be less vulnerable if detained in local authority accommodation. I am not sure this is so. Some people may well feel less intimidated, but would they all be provided with adequate standards of care, be given protection from other detained persons, and be provided with appropriate medical and legal advice? Would local authorities provide such standards, bearing in mind current financial restraints? And if so would things change all that much? In one sense detention is still detention whether the custodians are in uniform or not. My own view is that it may in the long run be more important to re-examine the service provisions, including the link between the police and the social worker and medical professions, than be too concerned about the place of safety. Were services to be improved other improvements might follow.

The Subjects in their Social Setting

Research undertaken on Section 136 has been comparatively rare. At first it was conducted almost entirely by psychiatrists, but lately has included sociologists. Three large projects undertaken by MIND have looked at the manner in which the police use police stations as a place of safety and the police contacts with the psychiatrists in the mental hospitals (Rogers and Faulkner, 1987; Rassaby, Rogers and Faulkner, 1989; Bean *et al.*, 1989). Unlike almost all other research on Section 136 the MIND studies examined the interactions between the police and the subject and the police and the psychiatrist. They give important new data on the way the police deal with difficult and varied groups of people. They show, too, the way the police, a semi-profession, have to negotiate and fare with a more established profession (see particularly Rogers, 1989).

Consider first some of the socio-demographic features of those detained. Much of the earlier research had tended to show that males predominated over females in Section 136 referrals — as did the MIND Stage I study (166 males to 107 females: Rogers and Faulkner, 1987). Stages II and III, however, reported a more even balance, with Stage III reporting 50 males and 50 females (Rassaby *et al.*, 1989; Bean *et al.*, 1989). In Stages II and III of the MIND study all referrals were included rather than those subsequently admitted to the hospitals. Even so these would not have accounted for the differences. Perhaps a new trend is being discovered, or perhaps chance factors are operating.

Next, consider the ages of those detained and where they lived. Most of the earlier research findings show that the referrals (or patients) were young, i.e. under 35 years of age. The MIND studies tend to confirm this; here, if anything, slightly more were in the younger age group. In terms of accommodation and home conditions earlier research suggested that London acts as a 'sump' attracting drifters and itinerants from other parts of the country. Section 136 individuals were such drifters and itinerants. Some subjects in the MIND study certainly were, but most were not. Those who were homeless — and a substantial number were without a settled address — may have given the impression of being wanderers. Yet when we looked more closely, these subjects were attached to a geographical area with friends, family and acquaintances there. Our evidence shows these subjects had often been detained before on Section 136, and if not by the same policeman then certainly at the same police station. In other words, they belonged to a certain area and remained close to it — and were not new arrivals in the London area. They were attached to a certain geographical area, with family, friends or acquaintances in that area.

In the light of the above it is no surprise, therefore, to see that so few subjects were employed at the time of their detention: some studies give data of around 7 per cent employed, the MIND study gives 15 per cent; and no surprise, either, to see that most come from social classes 4 and 5.

Table 1   Ethnic grouping of patients in Stage III MIND study *

Ethnic Grouping	Frequency	%
Afro-Caribbean	33	36.3
Asian	4	4.4
White European	47	51.6
Others + Not Known	7	7.7
TOTAL	91	100.0

*I am grateful to MIND for granting permission for the Table to be reproduced.

Table 1 shows the ethnic group of patients as taken from Stage III of the MIND study (Bean *et al.*, 1989). The matter of ethnicity has been mentioned before. The data for Table 1 shows the majority of subjects to be white/caucasian but the high proportion of Afro-Caribbeans found in this and other studies is a feature of Section 136 referrals generally: this in contrast to the relatively low proportion of Asians. The percentages of Afro-Caribbeans, however, vary: the Stage I report found 18 per cent Afro-Caribbean, but the Stage II report found 50 per cent. However, both show an under-representation of the Asian group.

There may be many reasons for an over-representation of Afro-Caribbeans in this and other research studies on Section 136. But as yet we can only speculate, for no one seems to know. My view is that this type of deviance amongst mentally disordered blacks is simply more visible: that is, it takes place on the streets. If so, one could then postulate a labelling type argument: i.e., when the police detain the individual, he/she acts out the label and a further process of detention ensues based on what Scheff calls 'the nature of uncertainty' inherent in all psychiatric diagnosis. Social workers and psychiatrists confirm the label (Scheff, 1964). Thus a process starts and ends which serves mainly to confirm stereotypes. But this, too, is speculation; a more detailed study is overdue. There may also be a social class component to consider: our data shows an over-representation of white subjects in social classes 4 and 5, and Afro-Caribbeans, as opposed to Asians, are more likely to be in social classes 4 or 5 generally.

To return to and summarize the data: research findings show that the modal type of person detained by the police under Section 136 was young (under 35 years of age), single, homeless or perhaps wandering or living in temporary accommodation. Most were ethnically white but with an over-representation of Afro-Caribbean blacks.

Subjects' Contact with Police and Police Contact with Psychiatrists

Data given here on the police involvement with the subjects and their subsequent removal to a place of safety is taken from the MIND research which shows a process operating something like this (Bean *et al.*, 1989). The process starts when a member of the public notifies the police that an individual is behaving strangely; sometimes, perhaps, in a threatening way. The police then deal with what is seen by them as a public disturbance. Mostly this occurs in the early or late evening, though a few occurrences are between 9.00 a.m. and 5.00 p.m. The incidents themselves are often frightening to the members of the public for they are not incidents where the individual is behaving simply in a bizarre way, or being mildly amusing. Rather, the incidents tend to be perceived as serious, with members of the public saying they are frightened by the person's behaviour (for he/she is sometimes involved in and perpetrates rather high levels of personal violence). The data in the MIND study shows that sometimes neighbours and others have put up with such behaviour over a fairly long period of time — five or six hours was not uncommon (Bean *et al.*, 1989).

This first stage shows that the police respond to calls from other people to deal with an incident. Dealing with an incident also means 'doing something' about it. In effect this means arresting the individual and/or removing him/her from that immediate vicinity. To pursue this point for a moment: the pressure on the police to act or 'do something' should not be dismissed too readily. The police have to consider their image, their public relations and the effects on the public if they were to leave the person unattended. Indeed, with hindsight, often there seem many good reasons why they should have acted. The MIND research, along with other studies, shows that these persons are 'more ill' or 'more seriously disturbed' than the usual mental hospital referral (Bean *et al.*, 1989). The subsequent psychiatric diagnoses list a high proportion of them as schizophrenics of one type or another, or as suffering from an affective psychosis, with an equally large number diagnosed as suffering from a personality disorder. Another group — about one third — were said to have had a serious psychotic episode of some sort — though no specific diagnosis was given (*ibid.*, 1989).

The first phase, then, is about the police being called by a member of the public. To the police, psychiatric disturbances are also social disturbances — it is doubtful if they would bother to deal with a psychiatric disturbance which was not also a social one. A person deemed to be psychiatrically ill, but not creating a social disturbance, would not draw police attention: the police interest is not on the medical/welfare condition of the individual, but on the public order and the repercussions on public order where controls are required. Nor does it appear that the police go looking for psychiatrically ill individuals. The police almost always approached the person as if they were dealing with an offender who had committed or was about to commit an offence (Rogers, 1989). Only later, when he/she was in the police van or at the police station, did they consider dealing with him/her as mentally disordered. In a few cases it seems the individual's behaviour was so bizarre that it was obvious he/she was mentally disordered, but this was the exception. This finding is not easy to explain. One would have thought mental disorder of this magnitude was easy to recognize. But it seems that the police were not prepared for a mentally disordered person (relatively few deal with Section 136 cases). The police appear to be more geared up to expect and cope with a disruptive offender. And presumably, too, the range of behaviour they see is such as to make them less aware of eccentricity, or perhaps they learn to ignore it altogether. Either way these persons appeared to the police to be offenders first and as mentally disordered later.

The second phase involves the police with the psychiatrists and social workers — professionals and semi-professionals. A draft Code of Practice provided by the DHSS gives the procedures to be adopted and the expectations of the various parties involved. It says 'the police officer has powers to take a person found in a public place, apparently suffering from mental disorder, and in immediate need of care and control, to a place of safety'. Moreover, 'health authorities, social service authorities and the police should make arrangements to collaborate in the use of that power and the necessary consequential arrangements' (DHSS, 1988). In fact no such contact with social workers occurred. Rarely were they called by the police, and if they were they did not come out to see the detained person. When the police took the person to a mental hospital — itself a place of safety — social workers were not called there either. In fact they were ignored by both groups, playing no part in the proceedings. It is not easy to explain why this should be so.

The main question to be asked, however, is 'Does collaboration exist between the various professional groups?' Here we must rely on data from the MIND study to answer the question — and of course only be concerned with the police and the psychiatrists. Collaboration was defined as involving professionals working together sharing knowledge and experience. Under such conditions, status divisions would be reduced to a minimum with a frank and open exchange of views. Also there would be a feeling of mutual worth underpinning the way group members acted towards each other. Collaboration, clearly a hallmark of professional acceptance, was defined as having the following indicators: reduction in status divisions, frankness and openness, and feelings of mutual worth' (Bean *et al.*, 1989).

Dealing first with a reduction in status division: the MIND study shows the police were often the supplicants asking for a patient to be admitted to the mental hospital rather than colleagues working with a psychiatric team. In the MIND research, the evidence shows how the police were often kept waiting at the hospitals for over an hour, and occasionally for over three hours, to be seen by the psychiatrists. On one occasion involving an inordinately long wait, the police officer said he had 'to press the psychiatrist into doing something for the person'. On another occasion when the police officer was kept waiting for over four hours, he felt additionally aggrieved when a nurse blamed the whole matter on him. ' "She said it was the bloody police's fault the person was brought to the hospital. She didn't take into account the fact that somebody called us in the first place'' ' (Rogers, 1989).

Many psychiatrists confirmed that the police were kept waiting at the hospital, but they saw nothing wrong in this, or they justified their practice in some way. One psychiatrist said he asked the police to wait because he could not guarantee the detained persons' admission. Another said he kept the police waiting as he might have required assistance with a violent patient. And another said, 'The police should have telephoned in advance before bringing in the patient. This patient was a well known black-listed person. So it was a waste of time bringing him here' (Rogers, 1989). Incidentally this comment illustrates again the extent of confusion about Section 136, with the psychiatrists seeing it as an admission order.

On matters concerning the reduction in status divisions, consider the extent of feedback given to the police. Again, taking the data from the MIND research, the psychiatrists were asked if they informed the police on the outcome of the interviews, and more than half said they had. However, when looked at more closely, it turned out there were only four instances where the psychiatrists directly informed the police. The police were certainly informed but mostly by others such as nursing staff, the detained individuals, or someone else. Occasionally, the police were told that the person would be admitted, and were present when it happened, but more likely they said they handed him/her over and rang a few days later to find out the result (*ibid.*, 1989).

Next, on the question of frankness and openness, the police said their views were often discounted. Sometimes, they were not invited to comment on the individual's mental state, and often not expected to give details of the incidents leading to the person's detention. It was as if they had no function other than 'fetchers and carriers' for the psychiatrists. On the question of 'a feeling of mutual worth', the psychiatrists were asked about the ways they viewed the police. Rarely did they believe they had a good relationship with the police in spite of a recognition of what one called 'a mutual dependency'. Many objected to the way the police 'were too eager to dump the social problem on to the hospital'. Yet one psychiatrist said, 'We try to get on. The police try harder than us. But that's because the psychiatrists don't have to try' (quoted in Bean *et al.*, 1989).

In spite of these rather disparaging views most psychiatrists thought the police were the appropriate occupational group to operate Section 136. But again, and using the MIND data, approval of the police was less than it seemed. Psychiatrists saw the police as the only group who would do that dirty work. They saw the police as being in the first line, unable to believe any other occupational group could do their work. Some psychiatrists saw the police as having a duty to maintain the peace, which would inevitably bring them in contact with such individuals. Occasionally, psychiatrists demanded more training for the police — but mostly the police were seen as the right group for Section 136 if only because no one else would do it (Bean *et al.*, 1989).

The psychiatrists also thought most referrals were appropriate. Indeed, there seemed to be a sort of inevitability about most of them. 'I don't see what else the police could have done,' said one psychiatrist; and another said, 'The patient had been violent, smashing up windows, and had a previous admission to hospital,' adding, 'What else could one do?' When referrals were 'inappropriate' it was because individuals were 'not ill' or 'not a danger to themselves or others, nor was their condition severe enough to warrant admission'. Sometimes the referral was 'appropriate' although misgivings were added: 'only appropriate because patient was a known nutter,' or, 'probably appropriate, the patient has been sick for years and is increasingly damaging property' (*ibid.*, 1989). Yet curiously enough the psychiatrists distinguished between 'making appropriate referrals' and 'being able to recognize mental disorder.' Whereas the police were thought to be competent at the first, they were not so regarded at the second. Moreover, when they were also asked 'were the police competent at handling mentally disordered people?' the same number of psychiatrists said they were not, or expressed uncertainty about it (*ibid.*, 1989).

What seemed to be happening was that the psychiatrists distinguished between individual police actions, of which they usually approved, and the position of the police as a social group, of which they usually did not approve. So, whilst individual police were seen as being able to recognize mental disorder, or handle it, the police as a social group were regarded with less approval. This seems to suggest that 'collaboration' as defined here rarely existed, and the expectations in the Draft Code of Practice remain unfulfilled.

Implications of the Research

The research data reviewed here on Section 136 suggests the police are required to deal with a group of subjects who, amongst other things, are socially disruptive, often displaying florid psychiatric symptoms. The data also shows that the police, in seeking help and control of this group, often meet with a rather implacable medical profession less than eager to accord them appropriate professional recognition. The police are reduced to the level of supplicants and placed in a subordinate role. These findings, which to an outsider may show attitudes which are petty and unseemly and likely to harm the subject, seem to demonstrate a long standing dispute between the two groups. The police see the psychiatrists as refusing to admit mentally disordered individuals without parading their professional dominance. In contrast the psychiatrists see the police as coming close to usurping their position as the sole profession with the right to diagnose and treat the mentally disordered. And so the battle lines are drawn.

We ought not to believe that Section 136 is likely to fade away, although primary health care systems could be developed which reduce police involvement. More likely the trend is towards greater police activity. It is clear from the programmes of community based mental health services that deinstitutionalization results in more contact between the police and mentally disordered people. Often deinstitutionalization means the absence of primary health care thereby forcing the police into the front line. This makes it all the more important that police act appropriately in dealing with the mentally disordered and there is proper liaison between police and other services. The MIND research shows that we can look in vain for assistance from the social services departments; they were ignored by police and psychiatrists, nor did they show any interest in being otherwise (Bean *et al.*, 1989).

As far as the police were concerned the MIND research shows they were an efficient source of referral, being able to select persons regarded by the psychiatrists as mentally disordered. However, they were not given the professional recognition they deserved. As matters stand there are few opportunities for the police to develop skills with the mentally disordered, and anyway it is too easy to demand better training when there is nothing to suggest that training will produce direct returns. The police will still come up against the impervious medical/psychiatric profession secure behind their institutional bulwarks, able to decide whether patients should or should not be admitted. One wonders how long the police will continue to use Section 136, preferring perhaps to charge the individual with an offence and leave the court to decide. If so, the effect on the prison system would be profound.

At the wider policy level the question is how to equip primary health care systems with the means to identify the mentally disordered and reduce pressure on the police to intervene. Community based assessment facilities would be an answer, but given the current financial political climate one should not rely on this being developed. Perhaps GPs could make a greater contribution, but doubts remain there too. Realistically, the police will continue to operate against a backdrop of hospital closures, and presumably continue to be involved in professional rivalry, for there is little to suggest the medical profession will change.

References

BEAN, P. T. (1980) *Compulsory Admissions to Mental Hospitals*, Chichester, Wiley.

BEAN, P. T. (1986) *Mental Disorder and Legal Control*, Cambridge, Cambridge University Press.

BEAN, P. T., RASSABY, E., ROGERS, A. and FAULKNER, A. (1989) *Arrangements for Treatment and Care*, London, MIND.

BERRY, C. and ORWIN, A. (1966) 'No fixed abode', *British Journal of Psychiatry*, 112, pp. 1019–25.

BUTLER REPORT (1975) *Report of the Committee on Mentally Abnormal Offenders*, Cmnd 6244, London, HMSO.

HOME OFFICE (1975) *Home Office Consolidated Circular to the Police on Crime and Kindred Matters*, London, HMSO.

KELLEHER, M. and COPELAND, J. (1972) 'Compulsory psychiatric admissions by the police', *Medicine, Science and the Law*, 12, 3, p. 220.

MOUNTNEY, G., FRYERS, T. and FREEMAN, H. L. (1969) 'Psychiatric emergencies in an urban borough', *British Medical Journal*, 1, pp. 478–500.

RASSABY, E., ROGERS, A. and FAULKNER, A. (1989) *A Public Face*, London, MIND.

ROGERS, A. (1989) *Psychiatric Referrals from the Police*, Unpublished Ph.D Thesis, University of Nottingham.

ROGERS, A. and FAULKNER, A. (1987) *A Place of Safety*, London, MIND.

SCHATZMAN, L. and STRAUSS, A. (1966) 'A sociology of psychiatry: A perspective and some organising foci', *Social Problems*, 14, 1.

SCHEFF, T. (1964) *Being Mentally Ill*, New York, Aldine.

SIMS, A. and SYMONDS, R. L. (1975) 'Psychiatric referrals from the police', *British Journal of Psychiatry*, 127, pp. 171–8.

Notes on Contributors

Pamela Abbott is a senior lecturer in sociology and social policy at Polytechnic South West (Plymouth) and has written in the areas of health, health inequalities, mental handicap, health visiting, biopolitics and women and social class, as well as authoring a textbook on feminist sociology (with Claire Wallace).

Philip Bean is a senior lecturer in the department of social policy and administration, University of Nottingham. Prior to that he worked as research officer for the Medical Research Council. His interests are in the field of criminology and mental health, where he has published widely. His chapter in this volume describes part of a larger study undertaken by MIND with the cooperation of the Police Foundation, an account of which was published by MIND in 1989.

Maria Lorentzon came to Britain in the early 1960s, where she qualified as a nurse and midwife in London. In the 1970s she commenced the study of social science at the Polytechnic of North London and later at the London School of Economics, where she was awarded a Ph.D. for research into nursing and social work. She has spent most of her working life within the National Health Service and is currently employed by the North East Thames Regional Health Authority, coordinating nursing research and quality assurance. Her academic interests include the sociology of professions and the exploration of the image of nursing.

David McCallum teaches at the University of Technology, Melbourne, Australia. His research interests include historical perspectives on social policy, and a forthcoming book on the role of psychology in the development of the Australian school system will be published in England by Falmer Press.

Lesley Mackay is currently a senior research fellow in the department of sociology, University of Lancaster. She is working on an ESRC-funded project, 'Inter-professional relations in health care'. Her book *Nursing a Problem* was published by Open University Press in 1989.

Fraser McLellan is an Information and Research Officer for Leeds Health Authority.

Des McNulty lectures in sociology at Glasgow College. His main interests are in political and industrial sociology.

Roger Sapsford is a lecturer in research methods at the Open University. As well as contributing to courses on methods, social psychology, criminology and social policy, he has carried out research on life-sentence and other prisoners, mothers of mentally handicapped children, and women and social class.

Michael Sheppard is a senior lecturer in social work at Polytechnic South West (Plymouth). His current research interest is the work of community psychiatric nurses and social workers. He is author of a number of papers on social work and a monograph on child abuse. His book *Mental Health: the role of the approved social worker* was published by University of Sheffield Press in 1990, and another, *Mental Health Work in the Community: social work and community psychiatric nursing*, is to be published by Falmer Press.

Roger Sibeon is a lecturer in the department of social work studies, University of Liverpool. He is author of a number of papers on social policy and social work. His current research interest is in the sociology of social work, and this interest is reflected in his contribution to Martin Davies (Ed.) *Sociology of Social Work* (1989).

Claire Wallace is a senior lecturer in sociology and social policy at Polytechnic South West (Plymouth). She has published mainly in the area of youth, family and work and is an author of a textbook on feminist sociology (with Pamela Abbott).

Author Index

Subject Index

academic nursing, 34–5, 38, 91, 99–100

Association of Teachers in Social Work Education, 98–100

Association of the Directors of Social Services, 94, 98–100

ancillary workers, 45

Barclay Report (1982), 54, 56, 60, 61, 63, 64, 68

Briggs Report (1972), 54, 55, 56, 57, 60, 63, 127

Butler Report (1975), 158

British Association of Social Workers, 91, 97, 98–100

British Medical Association (BMA), 44, 45

career, 31

carers/care/caring, 20, 25, 26, 27, 34, 35, 38, 48, 64, 68, 69, 132

case work, 13, 14, 15, 68, 101, 104, 112–19, 124

Central Council for the Education and Training of Social Work, 5, 15, 91, 94, 98–103

Certificate of Qualification in Social Work (CQSW), 98–103

charity, 11, 60, 112, 137

Charity Organisations Society, 11, 12, 13, 90, 117

child/children, 14, 30, 31, 61, 113, 117, 118, 120–28, 130, 135, 136, 141, 142, 143, 144, 145

child abuse/battering/neglect, 6, 16, 64, 71, 147

Childrens Act (1948), 14

childbirth, 18

childcare facilities, 30, 31

childhood, 13–15

Children and Young Persons Act 1963, 15

class, 3, 24, 113, 128, 131, 135, 137, 140, 147, 160, 161,

client, 1, 3, 6, 7, 25, 26, 74–8, 81, 83, 84, 85, 97, 98, 104, 117, 123, 130, 148

community, 67, 69, 76, 78, 84, 127

community care, 64, 67, 154

community social work, 76

community work, 25, 126

control (of clients), 3, 26, 36, 60, 61, 71, 125, 131, 132, 133, 134, 148, 166

control (of professionals), 8, 49, 101, 102

Court Report on Child Health (1976), 127

crime/criminal, 10, 61

Cumberledge Report on Community Nursing (1986), 127, 130,

discourse, 8, 10, 16, 17, 83, 120–21, 133, 134, 135, 136, 138, 139, 144–6

doctors/General Practitioners, 5, 16, 17, 83, 123–5, 129, 132, 134, 147, 166

Dr. Barnado, 11, 13

education, 5, 34, 35, 38, 51, 53, 64, 68, 70, 82

ethnic division, 3, 24, 78, 123, 129, 156, 157, 160, 161

family, 5, 10–17, 20, 30, 53, 68, 80–1, 113, 117, 120–47

feminism/feminist, 3, 10, 53, 132, 135, 146

Florence Nightingale, 17, 20, 21, 22, 32, 54, 60, 142